Heart Attack!

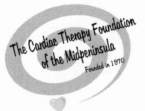

The Cardiac Therapy Foundation of the
Midpeninsula, founded in 1970 in Palo Alto,
California, is a unique cardiac rehabilitation
program, currently owned and operated by the
heart attack patients themselves. Its well-qualified
staff provides a full range of assistance, including
exercise classes, social support, stress reduction groups,
nutritional counseling, and health education. The
Foundation has helped thousands of heart attack
patients to lead healthier, longer, and more
vibrant lives.

HEART ATTACK!

Advice for Patients by Patients

Kathleen Berra
Gerald W. Friedland
Christopher Gardner
Francis H. Koch
Donna Louie
Nancy Houston Miller
Robin Wedell

with

Barton Thurber

YALE UNIVERSITY PRESS   *New Haven and London*

The information and suggestions contained in this book are not intended to replace the services of your physician or caregiver. Because each person and each medical situation is unique, you should consult your own physician to get answers to your personal questions, to evaluate any symptoms you may have, or to receive suggestions on appropriate medications.

The authors have attempted to make this book as accurate and up-to-date as possible, but it may nevertheless contain errors, omissions, or material that is out of date at the time you read it. Neither the authors nor the publisher have any legal responsibility or liability for errors, omissions, out-of-date material, or the reader's application of the medical information or advice contained in this book.

Set in the Stone Clan types by Tseng Information, Durham, North Carolina. Printed in the United States of America by Vail-Ballou Press, Binghamton, New York.

Library of Congress Cataloging-in-Publication Data

Heart attack : advice for patients by patients / Kathleen Berra . . . [et al.].
   p. cm.
   Includes bibliographical references and index.
   ISBN 0-300-08980-5 (cloth : alk. paper)—
   ISBN 0-300-09190-7 (pbk. : alk. paper)
   1. Myocardial infarction—Popular works.   I. Berra, Kathy.
RC685.I6 H425 2001
616.1′237—dc21   2001033256

A catalogue record for this book is available from the British Library.

∞ The paper in this book meets the guidelines for permanence and durability of the Committee on Production Guidelines for Book Longevity of the Council on Library Resources.

10 9 8 7 6 5 4 3 2 1

*In loving memory
of Jerry Fox, a
man of ideas*

Contents

Part III The Health Professionals' Perspectives

Preface

Jerry Fox and Jacob Gershon

About seven years ago, four of us (Jerry Fox, Jacob Gershon, Max Kramer, and David Moses) who were participants in a cardiac rehabilitation program realized that a book about heart attack, written by people who had had them, could not only be unique, but might inspire and educate millions throughout the world. It could be helpful even to those who had not had a heart attack but were eager to prevent one. After we decided to go ahead, some reluctance set in about placing our personal medical histories in the public realm. The proposal languished until we realized that by using pseudonyms (as we have done) we could protect our own privacy and that of those close to us.*

We also felt we needed a solid scientific groundwork for any such discussion. So we asked eight well-qualified professionals to write chapters on heart attack, treatment, nutrition, and guidelines for choosing an effective program, as well as a chapter on cardiac rehabilitation in action. (If you would like more information on any of these topics, see the Notes at the back of the book. None of the references cited there require specific medical training. A Glossary provides help with any difficult medical terms.) The reader will find that some scientific material is covered more than once. We decided to retain this overlap for two reasons: the material addressed is literally a matter of

---

* The widow and children of one participant requested that we use his true name (Jerry Fox), as he has now passed away and there is no further need to protect his medical history. We are happy to oblige.

life and death, and each author has a unique slant on what may at first seem familiar. All of the professionals who wrote chapters checked the contributions of the participants for scientific accuracy and made changes as appropriate.

The normal values of blood pressure, cholesterol, blood fats, and sugar are indicated in the chapters written by the medical professionals. To avoid confusing the reader, each author has used values based on the National Cholesterol Education Panel III, published in 2001, and other national guidelines. The new guidelines for cholesterol apply to persons with clinical coronary artery disease, symptomatic carotid artery disease, peripheral arterial disease, abdominal aortic aneurysm, and diabetes, and to persons without these diseases.

About half of this book was contributed by participants in cardiac rehabilitation programs. In that respect it differs significantly from the otherwise excellent books on cardiac rehabilitation, all of which have been written by doctors and nurses. We offer the perspective of those who have had angina or a heart attack and have lived to tell the story. Their message is universal and mirrors the experience of anyone living wherever heart attacks are common (although, obviously, the stories mirror the circumstances of the individuals' lives).

Each participant you will encounter here has a unique tale. Yet you will also find a considerable commonality, especially in the ways they have come to value their own cardiac rehabilitation program. Each story has also been selected to make one or more important points about heart attacks, recovery, and rehabilitation.

One of the striking features of the participants' stories is how many have survived and are doing well long after they started experiencing angina or had a heart attack; two, in fact, have survived thirty years or longer. New participants find that meeting these people and hearing their stories is uplifting and gives them hope. We have included as many stories as possible—for the insight they provide into what to expect in the future, and so that the reader can see what is required for a satisfactory long-term outcome. The disadvantage of this approach is that some participants describe coronary angiography, bypass surgery, and clotbuster therapy as new and experimental procedures. They are thinking of their own experiences of decades ago. Currently each procedure is routine, well established, and safe.

In addition, heart attack patients once spent a much longer time in the hospital than they do today. Physicians did not allow their patients to return to work or begin cardiac rehabilitation for many months after the heart attack. But if you have had a recent heart attack, we hope you will feel fortunate that you probably spent a short time in the hospital, were able to return to work quickly, and were referred early to cardiac rehabilitation. In this spirit, after Chapter 1 on heart attack basics, we begin our participants' accounts with the most contemporary story (Chapter 2), to show what happens to cardiac patients in the new millennium. We follow this with another contemporary story in Chapter 3, which differs from the previous tale in that the heart attack victim devised his own cardiac rehabilitation program.

Chapter 4 discusses the importance of teamwork, both among medical practitioners and between the patient and his or her medical team.

Chapters 5 through 7 present three people who describe the different ways they managed to prevent angina from progressing to a heart attack.

Chapters 8 and 9 discuss two ways to reverse coronary artery disease after a heart attack or bypass surgery.

After that, Chapters 10 and 11 tell stories that fly in the face of the perceived wisdom that heart attacks do not occur in the young, for example, or in women (at least not as often as they occur in men). They can. They do.

What follows in Chapter 12 is a discussion of factors that put a person at risk for a heart attack, once again from the patient's point of view.

Each contributor describes his or her medical history; some

describe what happens physically and emotionally when a heart attack occurs, and some describe, in dramatic detail, what open-heart surgery feels like, before the procedure as well as afterward.*

Some contributors had problems with the diagnosis of their illness, or of other medical problems that occurred simultaneously. We have not included these accounts to frighten you or make you mistrust your doctor, for all of the writers realize that doctors do the very best they can, but sometimes the diagnosis is by no means obvious. You may exhibit an unusual combination of symptoms, or your doctor may be reluctant to order what appear to be unnecessary and expensive tests. These are part and parcel of the modern practice of medicine; we emphasize that all of us have the highest regard for our own physicians and recognize that they are doing a wonderful job on our behalf. Where there are problems, diagnostic or otherwise, we have tried always to indicate potential solutions as well, so that if you find yourself in similar circumstances you will have a sense of what to do next.

No matter where you live, whether you have had a heart attack or not, whether you are in a cardiac rehabilitation program or not, we hope the stories here will educate and inspire you to heart health and, if you have had a heart attack, to recovery.

Most of our professionals and participants agreed to be interviewed by Gerald Friedland and told their stories orally. Barton Thurber then put them into a uniform format. Sonny Adams, Francis Koch, and Max Kramer wrote their chapters themselves. Gerald Friedland also made some suggestions that were incorporated in Chapter 13.

* For the reader interested in looking at these stories in chronological order, from the most recent episode of heart attack or angina to the earliest, that order is as follows: 2000, Chapters 2 and 3; 1995, Chapter 11; 1988, Chapter 4; 1985, Chapter 6; 1984, Chapter 8; 1981, Chapters 9 and 12; 1974, Chapter 5; 1966, Chapter 10; and 1965, Chapter 7.

We are all most grateful to Kevin Murphy, administrative associate in the Stanford University Department of Radiology, who typed (and retyped!) the entire manuscript; to Jean Thomson Black and Margaret Otzel of Yale University Press for their help and encouragement; to Vivian Wheeler for her editorial services; and to Miriam Friedland for donating her automobile to the Cardiac Therapy Foundation of the Midpeninsula, Palo Alto, California—a gift that enabled this project to go forward.

All of the proceeds from *Heart Attack!* will be donated to the Cardiac Therapy Foundation of the Midpeninsula, a nonprofit organization and one of the first community-based cardiac rehabilitation programs in the United States.

PART I

Heart Attack Basics

CHAPTER 1

Heart Attack and You

Kathleen Berra and Gerald W. Friedland

Did you know that, worldwide, twenty-three people each minute have a heart attack? This adds up to about 12 million heart attacks a year. More than 1 million Americans will have a heart attack each year, and 14 million Americans now living have had a heart attack or angina.[1] In fact, if you live in an industrialized country, heart disease is either the number one killer there or a major cause of death.

Even when heart disease does not kill, it maims, so if you have had a heart attack, you may well find yourself attending a cardiac rehabilitation program to help in your recovery. If you do, remember that millions of people just like you are in similar programs all over the world.

But there is also good news: your chances of dying from a heart attack grow less and less. In fact, the United States Centers for Disease Control and Prevention, in Atlanta, Georgia, report that in the past fifty years there has been a stunning 60 percent reduction in mortality from heart attacks.[2] If, for example, the death rate in 1963 from heart attacks had continued unchanged, an *additional* 621,000 Americans would have died in 1996 alone.

The Centers for Disease Control and Prevention found that this dramatic result was due in part to the systematic reduction of risk factors for heart attacks. In fact, if you have had a heart attack, one of the very best ways to learn how to reduce your risk factors is by enrolling in a cardiac rehabilitation program, which will provide a warm, nurturing, and supportive environment.

Fortunately, cardiac rehabilitation programs now exist wherever heart attacks are common, so if you have had a heart attack, help is likely to be at hand. If you happen to live in Western Europe, where the first such programs were established, probably you will automatically join a program after your heart attack. Other locations, unfortunately, lag behind Western Europe in this regard.

The goals and techniques of cardiac rehabilitation programs are similar all over the world, since they all follow similar published guidelines. (As you might expect, there are differences related to cultural and other factors, but the similarities between programs are far more significant than the differences.)

Unhappily, fewer than 40 percent of heart attack victims in the United States actually attend a cardiac rehabilitation program. In recognition of this statistic, a number of home-based rehabilitation programs are under way, in which the participant is monitored via telephone or by other means. These programs are discussed in detail in Chapter 16. Despite these ongoing efforts, many heart attack victims in the United States are not involved in any program, home based or not. Typically, these individuals construct their own, unmonitored rehabilitation program, which is why we have included one such story in this book (Chapter 3).

What Is a Heart Attack?

A heart attack occurs when an artery feeding blood to a section of heart muscle becomes completely blocked. If the blockage lasts long enough, the section involved will die. This process is called a heart attack, or myocardial infarction (MI). Scientists have discovered that when arteries are exposed to high levels of cholesterol, high blood pressure, high blood sugar, cigarette smoking, a diet high in saturated fats and cholesterol, and other risk factors, atherosclerosis often develops, followed by a process that results in blockage of the arteries and a heart attack if uncontrolled. The signs and symptoms of a heart attack should not be ignored; immediate medical care can, in some cases, restore blood flow and prevent permanent damage. In addition, the risk factors for heart disease (atherosclerosis) need to be aggressively managed to avoid developing disease in the heart arteries and throughout the body.

When someone has had a heart attack, the damage to the heart muscle is permanent. The best medicine can do is improve the patient's condition and help prevent a future heart attack or other heart problems. In addition, reducing risk factors for a heart attack also reduces the risk of a stroke. That is why it is crucial to know what factors put people at risk for a heart attack or a stroke in the first place—and what can be done to change these risk factors.[3]

Risk Factors

Typically, the risk factors for a heart attack and stroke include one or more of the following:

- Smoking or the use of other tobacco products
- High LDL "bad" cholesterol (levels greater than 100 mg/dL if you have atherosclerosis and/or diabetes)
- Low HDL "good" cholesterol (levels lower than 40 mg/dL)
- High triglycerides (levels greater than 150 mg/dL)
- High blood pressure (levels greater than 135/85 mm/Hg)
- Diabetes (high blood sugar levels, greater than 110 mg/dL)
- Sedentary lifestyle (exercising less than thirty minutes three or four times weekly) (Chapter 16)
- Obesity (being more than 20 percent over your ideal body weight or having a body mass index greater than 25)
- Negative emotional states (such as depression and/or high levels of anger and hostility) (Chapter 16)

- Lacking social support (being socially isolated)
- A diet high in saturated fat and lacking adequate plant-based foods such as nuts, grains, vegetables, and fruits (Chapter 13).

Here and in later chapters, we shall discuss these risk factors so that you can see how they influence your risk in and of themselves, and how they relate to greater risk when several occur together.

Smoking

Smoking affects the heart in many ways. A major cause of cancer and of diseases of the heart and lungs, it also blocks blood flow in the leg arteries. Particles of low-density lipoproteins (LDL) are very damaging to the artery walls. Smoking interferes with important actions of vitamin C, thereby allowing the LDL particles to become oxidized and even more damaging. Once oxidized, LDL particles generate an inflammatory reaction in the walls of the arteries, leading in turn to atherosclerosis. In addition, the nicotine in cigarette smoke can cause arteries, including the coronary arteries, to spasm (tighten up). The heart muscle will therefore receive less blood. Cigarettes also cause the blood pressure to go up, which increases the amount of work the heart has to do. And chronic high blood pressure leads to heart damage.

Other life-threatening complications of smoking include lung cancer and chronic obstructive pulmonary disease. Normally, oxygen and carbon dioxide are exchanged in the blood in air sacs within the lungs. With cigarette smoking, the walls of the air sacs break down; they become enlarged, and inadequate gas exchange results. This process is the notorious emphysema and it is not reversible. Once emphysema reaches a certain stage, individuals find themselves chronically short of breath even at low levels of physical activity. People with emphysema often have chronic bronchitis as well. The combination of chronic inflammation of the bronchial tubes and emphysema is known as chronic obstructive pulmonary disease (COPD). What is this like from the patient's point of view? Living with advanced COPD was absolute hell for Jerry Fox (Chapter 12); he found it "like being continuously tortured."

Smoking is by far the most serious risk factor for a heart attack. The best thing for smokers to do is to quit—the sooner the better. It is never too late to stop and it is crucial not to give up trying. Fortunately, nicotine replacements are available now, as well as new medications that make it easier than ever to stop smoking.

Quitting was easy for Verne Peters (Chapter 9), because he was extremely disciplined. For most people quitting is very difficult. Hans Forsell (Chapter 3) managed to reduce his smoking from two packs a day to one, but recent studies show you have to stop completely in order to derive any benefit at all. Some people require a major shock to quit: for Peter Jones (Chapter 6) it was the death from cancer of his father and many close friends. For David Moses (Chapter 7), who could not stop smoking for eleven years after developing angina, the shock was more personal: he developed cancer on the roof of his mouth. Jerry Fox (Chapter 12) had the most difficult time; he was hooked twice in his life by a cigarette offered at a party, once at age 24, then again at age 59. Each time he turned into a three-pack-a-day smoker. Consult the American Heart Association, the American Lung Association, the American Cancer Society (or the appropriate organization in the country in which you live), as well as your local cardiac rehabilitation program or your health care provider, for additional advice.

Elevated Cholesterol and Triglycerides

It is vital to regulate cholesterol levels. Everyone needs to know the results of their laboratory tests, including total cholesterol, LDL cholesterol, HDL cholesterol, and triglyceride levels.[4] Data collected from an enormous number of studies now irrefutably show that a person who has coronary artery disease or diabetes should make every effort to achieve at least the following levels:[5]

- Total cholesterol less than 200 mg/dL (5.2 mmol/L)
- LDL cholesterol less than 100 mg/dL (2.6 mmol/L)
- HDL cholesterol greater than 40 mg/dL (1.0 mmol/L), the higher the better
- Triglycerides less than 150 mg/dL (3.9 mmol/L); lower is probably even better (< 120 mg/dL).

There are many ways to achieve these levels, including exercise, diet, and weight loss. Some people are genetically inclined to produce too much cholesterol within their bodies, or are not able to clear it properly. New and truly excellent medicines are available to deal with these kinds of cholesterol problems. Regardless of the cause of the abnormal lipid values, weight control, appropriate nutrition, and exercise will benefit a person's health in remarkable ways in terms of heart disease, stroke, and certain cancers.

A number of other abnormalities are now emerging as potential risk factors. These include small, dense LDL particles; high levels of Lp(a), a particle with a protein called apo(a) stuck to its surface; high levels of an amino acid called homocysteine;[6] or high levels of a protein called highly sensitive C-reactive protein (CRP). Any number of these abnormalities can occur within the same person. Both Jacob Gershon (Chapter 8) and Sonny Adams (Chapter 10), for example, had high blood levels of homocysteine and Lp(a), together with small, dense LDL particles.

Small, dense LDL particles can pass easily through the arterial wall. There they are particularly susceptible to oxidation and can readily injure the arteries. They generally occur in the presence of high levels of triglycerides.

Elevated Lp(a) levels have an effect similar to that of elevated LDL cholesterol, but they also increase the likelihood of clot formation in blood vessels and can augment the risk of a heart attack. Your Lp(a) level is inherited, and if you have heart disease *and* a high Lp(a), you are potentially at high risk for a future heart attack and/or stroke. What we know today is that the best treatment for a high Lp(a) level is to keep your LDL and triglyceride levels as low as possible and your HDL level as high as possible.

Another new and interesting risk factor is a high homocysteine level. Researchers have found that a high level of homocysteine increases the susceptibility of arteries to developing atherosclerosis.

Elevated levels of highly sensitive C-reactive protein (measured in the blood as hs CRP) is also being carefully evaluated as a coronary risk factor. C-reactive protein indicates that an inflammatory process is occurring in the arteries, which appears to be related to an increased risk of a heart attack.

One of the problems with these emergent risk factors is that although data exist showing that they are related to the development of coronary artery disease and atherosclerosis in general, at present no data demonstrate unequivocally that changing levels of homocysteine, Lp(a), or hs CRP makes any difference in long-term outcomes.[7] Some few data indicate that increasing the size and buoyancy of the LDL particles can help prevent worsening atherosclerosis. Interestingly, the size of the LDL particle can be changed through weight control and dietary management to lower triglycerides below 120 mg/dL.

Current advice regarding the new factors is controversial. If you have a strong family history of coronary artery disease (especially if it has occurred in your father under the age of 55 or your mother under the age of 65), you might consider having yourself tested for these risk factors. The presence of these new risk factors was crucial in the cases of Jacob Gershon and Sonny Adams, both of whom had heart attacks early (Gershon at 51, Adams at 39), as well as a family history of coronary artery disease. If your homocysteine, Lp(a), or hs CRP levels are high, the decision about whether to try to lower them will be up to you and your doctor. The real point is to use the deepening knowledge of our body chemistry to minimize *all* risk factors for coronary artery disease.

If your homocysteine levels are high, consider taking a multivitamin tablet each day, one that contains 400 micrograms of folic acid.[8] If your levels are extremely high, your doctor may prescribe heavy doses of folic acid.

Niacin can lower Lp(a) in men and women, as can estrogen in women. Once again, however, only your own doctor can discuss the pros and cons of these treatments. The best way to increase LDL particle size and make the particles more buoyant (and less likely to cause atherosclerosis) is to lower triglycerides and keep HDL levels up. The lower the triglycerides, the larger and more buoyant the LDL particles will become.

Restricting intake of alcohol and simple sugars, losing weight if necessary, and regular exercise are outstanding ways to lower triglycerides and increase the size and buoyancy of LDL particles. Exercise, by the way, also helps to raise HDL levels. Both Jacob Gershon and Sonny Adams take folic acid for elevated homocysteine levels, and niacin for elevated Lp(a) levels and small dense LDL particles. Neither drinks alcohol, both avoid simple sugars, and both exercise regularly. Gershon, in addition, is on the Mediterranean diet (Chapter 13), which has raised his HDL levels and lowered his triglycerides.

High Blood Pressure

Lowering blood pressure to normal will dramatically decrease the chances of having a heart attack or stroke and will go a long way toward protecting the kidneys.[9]

Many Americans feel that a blood pressure of 135/85 and sometimes even higher is "okay." Often people will report that "140/90 is pretty good for me." If a person's blood pressure is in that range, it is *not* okay. It is *not* normal. The significance of a blood pressure in that range or higher cannot be overstated. It was a major risk factor for Hans Forsell (Chapter 3), Peter Jones (Chapter 6), and Jerry Fox (Chapter 12). To protect against heart attack and stroke, a person's blood pressure should be as close to 120/70 as possible. The best ways to decrease blood pressure are regular exercise, weight control, proper nutrition, salt restriction, and stress management. Many of us have all the tools needed to keep our blood pressure normal.

Fortunately, there are also many medicines that can help. Controlling blood pressure has been shown to dramatically reduce stroke and heart attack risk in all ages, including men and women in their seventies and eighties. It is never too late to help your heart and your brain by normalizing your blood pressure to 120/70. If you have high blood pressure, be sure to see your doctor. Medication is often a necessary addition to lifestyle management in order to control blood pressure.

Diabetes

Diabetes is especially dangerous for heart attack patients. The heart attack rate and the rate of death from heart attacks are four times higher in persons with diabetes than in those without.

There are two kinds of diabetes.[10] Persons with type 1 diabetes do not make insulin themselves and need insulin shots to survive. Their immune systems have destroyed the beta cells of the pancreas, which make insulin. Type 1 most often occurs in young persons and used to be called juvenile diabetes. However, it can also occur in adults. Type 2 is the more common type of diabetes. Insulin levels can be high, below normal, or normal; and the beta cells of the pancreas *do* continue to secrete insulin.

In 1955 about 2 percent of the general population in the United States had type 2 diabetes; 9 percent had type 2 diabetes in the year 2000. This enormous increase is related to both the increasing weight and the decreasing physical activity reported by American adults. Among Native Americans, Hispanic Americans, and African Americans, the rate is about 30 percent higher than in the general population. The problem is worldwide. Type 2 diabetes was rarely seen in young adults and children before the 1990s. Today it is much more common and is a major health threat to young people.

Type 2 diabetes affects two kinds of arteries in the body. The first site is the tiny arteries in the eyes or in the kidneys. If these arteries are affected, blindness or kidney failure can result. Second, type 2 diabetes can cause atherosclerosis in the larger arteries of the body. Jerry Fox (Chapter 12), for example, had type 2 diabetes and developed a high-grade blockage of the big artery on the left side of his neck, which supplies the left eye and the brain. To understand why, we need to look at the defects in the tissues that occur with this disease. These can arise in the muscles, in the beta cells of the pancreas, in the fat cells, and in the liver.

First, the muscle cells can become insulin resistant. Insulin functions to put glucose into the muscle cells, which is then used for energy. But if those muscles are resistant to insulin, the body has to secrete much more insulin to ensure that the normal amount of glucose gets into the muscles.

Second, the beta cells of the pancreas do not function well—or not well enough to secrete the very high levels of insulin required to overcome insulin resistance.

The third defect involves the fat cells, where the body stores most of its energy. When someone is not eating, the fat cells break up and release free fatty acids, which the muscles (including the muscles of the heart) can use for energy. In diabetes, this important process is not well regulated.

The final problem area in persons with type 2 diabetes is the liver, the main source of glucose in the body. If glucose is required, the liver produces it. If glucose is not required, the liver produces less. In type 2 diabetics, though, when the blood glucose levels go higher and higher, the liver does *not* stop making glucose.

All of these abnormalities of metabolism seen in diabetes result in abnormal levels of blood glucose. More important, if not treated, diabetes results in damage to vital organs—not only the eyes and the kidneys, but also the heart and the brain.

The most significant lifestyle changes a person can make to control type 2 diabetes are an appropriate diet, regular exercise, and weight control. Be sure to have your doctor check your blood glucose levels and refer you to a nutritionist if diabetes, even "borderline" diabetes, is found. The first treatment is life-style change. Fortunately, effective oral medications are available to help manage type 2 diabetes.

Obesity

Most people find that losing weight is very difficult. The benefits are enormous, though, especially if the weight is carried in the waist, so that they are shaped like an apple rather than a pear.[11]

There is a simple test for checking whether your weight is appropriate. Simply measure the largest circumference of your waist. In a man, that should not exceed 40 inches (102 cm); in a woman, it should not exceed 35 inches (89 cm). If your waist is equal to or larger than these measurements, your weight is concentrated in your abdomen. This is often called abdominal obesity, male-pattern fatness, or beer belly, and it can mean that you will be insulin resistant; likely to become a type 2 diabetic; and tend to have high blood pressure, high LDL levels, high triglycerides, and low HDL levels. All of these risk factors will put you at increased risk for a heart attack or stroke.

A far more accurate method for determining if you are overweight is the so-called body mass index, or BMI, which is the mathematical ratio between weight and height that correlates with body fat. The BMI can be calculated in three easy steps:

1. Multiply your weight in pounds by 703.
2. Multiply your height in inches by itself; that is, by your height in inches.
3. Divide the first product by the second.

Or find your BMI on the chart provided for you in this book (Table 1).[12] If you are using the metric system, you can calculate your BMI in just two steps:

1. Multiply your height in meters by itself; that is, by your height in meters.

Table 1. BMI based on weight in pounds and height in feet and inches.

Height Weight	5'0"	5'1"	5'2"	5'3"	5'4"	5'5"	5'6"	5'7"	5'8"	5'9"	5'10"	5'11"	6'0"	6'1"	6'2"	6'3"	6'4"
100	20	19	18	18	17	17	16	16	15	15	14	14	14	13	13	13	12
105	21	20	19	19	18	17	17	16	16	16	15	15	14	14	13	13	13
110	21	21	20	19	19	18	18	17	17	16	16	15	15	15	14	14	13
115	22	22	21	20	20	19	19	18	17	17	17	16	16	15	15	14	14
120	23	23	22	21	21	20	19	19	18	18	17	17	16	16	15	15	15
125	24	24	23	22	21	21	20	20	19	18	18	17	17	16	16	16	15
130	25*	25*	24	23	22	22	21	20	20	19	19	18	18	17	17	16	16
135	26	26	25*	24	23	22	22	21	21	20	19	19	18	18	17	17	16
140	27	26	26	25*	24	23	23	22	21	21	20	20	19	18	18	18	17
145	28	27	27	26	25*	24	23	23	22	21	21	20	20	19	19	18	18
150	29	28	27	27	26	25*	24	23	23	22	22	21	20	20	19	19	18
155	30	29	28	27	27	26	25*	24	24	23	22	22	21	20	20	19	19
160	31	30	29	28	27	27	26	25*	24	24	23	22	22	21	21	20	19
165	32	31	30	29	28	27	27	26	25*	24	24	23	22	22	21	21	20
170	33	32	31	30	29	28	27	27	26	25*	24	24	23	22	22	21	21
175	34	33	32	31	30	29	28	27	27	26	25*	24	24	23	22	22	21
180	35	34	33	32	31	30	29	28	27	27	26	25*	24	24	23	22	22
185	36	35	34	33	32	31	30	29	28	27	27	26	25*	24	24	23	23
190	37	36	35	34	33	32	31	30	29	28	27	26	26	25*	24	24	23
195	38	37	36	35	33	32	31	31	30	29	28	27	26	26	25*	24	24
200	39	38	37	35	34	33	32	31	30	30	29	28	27	26	26	25*	24
205	40	39	37	36	35	34	33	32	31	30	29	29	28	27	26	26	25*
210	41	40	38	37	36	35	34	33	32	31	30	29	28	28	27	26	26
215	42	41	39	38	37	36	35	34	33	32	31	30	29	28	28	27	26
220	43	42	40	39	38	37	36	34	33	32	32	31	30	29	28	27	27
225	44	43	41	40	39	37	36	35	34	33	32	31	31	30	29	28	27
230	45	43	42	41	39	38	37	36	35	34	33	32	31	30	30	29	28
235	46	44	43	42	40	39	38	37	36	35	34	33	32	31	30	29	29
240	47	45	44	43	41	40	39	38	36	35	34	33	33	32	31	30	29
245	48	46	45	43	42	41	40	38	37	36	35	34	33	32	31	31	30
250	49	47	46	44	43	42	40	39	38	37	36	35	34	33	32	31	30

2. Divide your weight in kilograms by the results of the first procedure. The BMI should not be greater than 25.

(Note that the BMI is inaccurate in competitive athletes, body-builders, pregnant women, lactating women, growing children, and frail or sedentary people.)

Diet and exercise help with weight loss and protect against diabetes, syndrome X (see Chapter 13), and heart disease. In most cases it is helpful to consult a nutritionist or weight-loss professional.

We urge everyone to make the lifestyle changes we have suggested, whether you have heart disease or not. You may be surprised at how much the *quality* of your life will improve. Your family and friends may also benefit, so set yourself on the path to a healthier, more vibrant life for all!

A Heart Attack or Not?

Suppose an apparently healthy person, living an apparently healthy life, suddenly develops chest pain or discomfort. How do we know if that chest pain is due to a heart attack or something else? [13]

The American Heart Association has developed guidelines to help with this question. Heart attack symptoms are the following:

- Uncomfortable pressure, fullness, squeezing, or pain in the center of the chest, lasting more than a few minutes.
- Pain spreading to the shoulders, neck, arms, elbows, wrists, fingers, somewhere around the shoulder blades, or the pit of the stomach.
- Chest discomfort with lightheadedness, fainting, sweating, nausea, or shortness of breath.

Any of these symptoms may result from a heart attack. When they occur, call your local emergency number or go immediately to the nearest emergency room.

Chest pain or discomfort, very much like what happens in a heart attack, can also occur and not be a heart attack. This pain, in the absence of an actual heart attack, is called *angina*. Its cause is a narrowing of the coronary arteries. It does not usually appear unless the heart is stimulated by exercise, emotional stress, exposure to very cold temperatures, or a large meal. During these situations the heart muscle needs more blood flow to be able to work harder. Only when the heart muscle does not get enough blood (because it is blocked by atherosclerosis) does the pain or discomfort occur.

The difference between a heart attack and angina is that angina comes and goes for two to five minutes, and is usually brought about by a stimulus such as the ones described above. It is quickly relieved by rest or by dissolving a nitroglycerine tablet under the tongue. The so-called three-tablet test is often used to distinguish angina from a heart attack: If one tablet is dissolved under the tongue every five minutes for fifteen minutes and the pain has not gone away after fifteen minutes, it is likely a heart attack. The emergency medical service should be contacted immediately.

Again, angina is more frequent after eating, during or after emotional stress, during cold weather, and with physical exertion. It can even wake up a sound sleeper, owing to a temporary spasm of the coronary arteries. This is known as vasospastic angina, or Prinzmetal angina, and is more common in heavy smokers and in young people.

Having angina does not necessarily mean you will have a heart attack. Helen L'Amoreaux (Chapter 5), for example, exercised vigorously for nineteen years, and during that entire period her angina did not progress. Amazingly, she then managed to eliminate the angina entirely by also going on a modified Ornish diet (Chapter 13). Peter Jones (Chapter 6) initially thought his angina was gas. Fortunately for him, his company had a preventive medicine program, and the company physician made the correct diagnosis in the nick of time. Sixteen years later he still has not had a heart attack, because the various treatments he received have prevented it. Finally, David Moses (Chapter 7) considers himself to be the bionic man because of the many procedures and devices he has received over the years. All of them together have prevented his angina—which began thirty-six years ago—from progressing into a full-blown heart attack.

If someone may be having a heart attack and calls an ambulance for transport to the hospital, paramedics in the ambulance on the way to the emergency room can obtain an electrocardiogram (EKG) and other measurements and transmit the results to the emergency room. Paramedics and emergency-room personnel are well equipped to handle the problems that can accompany a heart attack.

Pain in the chest that comes and goes in a few seconds, is a stabbing or shooting pain, or is localized to a spot the size of a coin, is unlikely to be either angina or a heart attack. Several tests can be performed to help determine if chest pain or unease is angina or something less serious, such as musculoskeletal discomfort or heartburn. One is a stress echo test, during which an EKG and a sonogram of the heart are obtained. The second test is for heart enzymes. When heart cells die, they release these enzymes into the blood; so if those levels are high, you have had a heart attack. If they are normal, you have probably not had a heart attack. Your physician may want to do an angiogram to determine more accurately if there are serious blockages. He or she will place a small catheter into an artery, perhaps in your groin, and image your heart arteries by means of a fluid visible on X-rays. This technique is very safe and allows for accurate measurement of artery size and the amount of atherosclerosis present (if any). It greatly helps in determining the appropriate method of care.

When It Is Not Your Heart

Many kinds of chest pain are due to diseases that do not actually involve the heart at all.[14] The stomach juices, which contain acid and pepsin, usually do not flow back up the esophagus. The sphincters at the lower end of the esophagus, and the inner lining of the esophagus itself, keep this from happening. If those mechanisms are deficient, though, stomach juices can flow backward in a phenomenon known as gastroesophageal reflux disease (GERD).

Reflux is often due to a hiatal hernia. Normally the tube that transports food from the mouth to the stomach—the esophagus—passes through a small hole in the diaphragm called the hiatus, before reaching the stomach, which lies beneath the diaphragm. In some people the hiatus enlarges, allowing part of the stomach to slide up into the chest. This permits the stomach acid to flow backward up the esophagus and can cause the discomfort often described as "heartburn" in the center of the chest.

It is usually easy to know if reflux is taking place or not. Timing is important: moderate to severe reflux usually happens after a big meal, typically a dinner party where rich, fatty foods, cocktails, wine and liqueur, coffee, and chocolates have been served. Citrus fruits and juices, and smoking, can also cause heartburn. Symptoms often begin later on, when bending down to take off one's shoes or lying in bed. Either or both can bring on acute heartburn. Antacids generally relieve the pain immediately.

Even doctors have difficulty distinguishing the milder forms of reflux from angina. A study about twenty-five years ago found that 40 percent of patients admitted to the hospital with a heart attack had had chest pain during the preceding period of three to four weeks—which was misdiagnosed as reflux. Jacob Gershon's chest pain, for example, was misdiagnosed as reflux for about a year (Chapter 8). Doctors, tests, and medications are today much more sophisticated, so difficulty in distinguishing heartburn from angina is less frequent.[15]

Intestinal problems can also be the culprits. Gas trapped in the left side of the colon, which is directly under the heart, can cause chest pain, as can stomach or duodenal ulcers, gallstones, or inflammation of the gallbladder.

Panic attacks sometimes generate symptoms of pain in the chest. People suffering from a panic attack feel extremely anxious. The heart may pound rapidly, they may experience sweating, shortness of breath, or difficulty in breathing, and feel dizzy or faint. If you have these types of symptoms, see a doctor to help deal with the attack and to ascertain that your heart is not the cause.

That a heart attack can sometimes mimic a panic attack is very important. When Jacob Gershon awoke late one night with chest pain, his wife called the doctor, who said he was having a panic attack. Actually, it was probably a heart attack.

A pulled or torn muscle in the chest wall due to vigorous coughing or strenuous exercise can cause chest pain with breathing. The pain is lessened by holding your breath. Pressing on the place where it hurts can be very painful.

Rib fractures and pleuritis (an inflammation·of the sac covering the lungs) can also cause chest pain. Your doctor can perform tests, such as chest X rays and blood tests, to differentiate these problems from heart-related pain.

It is crucial to remember that if there is any doubt at all, you should go to the nearest emergency room as soon as possible. If it turns out to be a false alarm, it is equally important not to feel embarrassed. Remember that a heart attack is a killer, and that delay can be deadly.

Understanding your own body's response to exercise, eating, and emotion can help you to know when to call your doctor for advice and when to go to the nearest emergency room if you experience chest pain. With patience, perseverance, and active participation, you can dramatically reduce your risk of a heart attack or stroke. Understanding and implementing lifestyle changes that will protect your heart and brain are critical to your longevity and quality of life. Working with your doctor to take the appropriate medications to lower your risk of a heart attack and stroke is also key to your continued good health.

The patients' tales in the chapters that follow will illustrate the material presented in this introductory chapter and in Part III.

PART II

The Participants' Perspectives

CHAPTER 2

A Heart Attack in the New Millennium

Jose Ibarra

January 17, 2000, began for me like any workday. I was up at 5:45 a.m., showered and had breakfast, was on the road by 7:50, and was in my office by 8:15.

I had booted up my laptop to check the weekend's e-mails when I started to feel weird and queasy, though not nauseated. I also had an uncomfortable tingly sensation in my jaws and along the triceps in both arms. I realized something was wrong and decided to wait a few moments to see what would happen. And, in fact, after a couple of minutes the sensations eased off.

All the same, I decided to take the day off. But because I felt something was not right, I wanted to get clearance from a medically trained person before driving home. At about 8:30 I called the clinic we have at work, but the voice-mail message told me that the nurse had not yet arrived; if there was an emergency, I should call our emergency number—which I did. The person answering told me not to move, that the emergency team would come immediately to my office. Not wanting to create an embarrassing commotion there, I said I would meet the team in the lobby.

I went down, and in a few moments five members of our emergency team arrived. They took my blood pressure and pulse, both of which were normal, and asked me detailed questions about what had happened. I told them I was still weak, but that I no longer had the tingling in my jaw or arms. They said there were two choices: they could take me directly to my doctor, or to the nurse's station. I chose the nurse, who by that time had arrived. After I repeated my story, she immediately called my doctor and secured an appointment for 11:00 that morning. She told me it was not safe to drive, so I called and asked my wife to pick me up.

When I arrived at the doctor's office, I still had no tingly sensations, but after recounting again what had happened, I said that I wanted to rule out a heart problem. He agreed and ordered an electrocardiogram (EKG).

The EKG technician was a jolly person and kidded me continuously. (For example, when I told him my age, he said I didn't look 59, so he would just put down 45.) I studied his face intently during the examination, because I knew that if he turned serious, I was in trouble.

Sure enough, he became very serious.

He told me to put my shirt on while he showed the results to my doctor. A moment later, the doctor hurried in and announced that I was, in fact, having a heart attack. He immediately called an ambulance and I was rushed to a nearby hospital.

In about an hour a cardiologist took a coronary angiogram, which showed that one of my coronary arteries was completely blocked. He performed an angioplasty and placed a stent in that artery, noting that all the other coronary arteries looked normal. He showed me before and after pictures of the affected artery, and even gave me copies of the angiogram to keep.

Almost everything that happened after this procedure was anticlimax. I did have some bleeding in the groin area where the catheter had been inserted, because the cardiologist had given me medication to prevent blood clots in the stent area. So the nurses applied a clamp, which pressed down to control the bleeding, and gave me a sleeping pill. I had a very restful night.

The rest of my recovery was uneventful, and I was discharged after three days.

Before being sent home, I was asked to look at a number of videos. The first piece of vital information I obtained was that the total cholesterol/HDL ratio is very important and needs to be 3 or less. To achieve this ratio requires a diet low in saturated fat, exercise, and appropriate medication. As it turned out, my total cholesterol at the time of my heart attack was 185 mg/dL (4.78 mmol/L) and my HDL was 37 mg/dL (0.96 mmol/L) so the ratio was 185/37 = 5, not 3 or less, which explained my cardiologist's prescription of a statin drug plus niacin to raise my HDL level. (He also prescribed aspirin to prevent clotting, and a beta-blocker.)

Another video was about stress as a risk factor for heart attack. I remember one patient in his early forties who had already had two bypass surgeries, despite a healthy diet, cholesterol-lowering drugs, and regular exercise after his first surgery. His cardiologist, however, remarked that he was still at risk for a heart attack and that unless he took steps to reduce his stress, he had only five or ten years to live. After learning meditation and reducing stress at work, his outlook changed, and his cardiologist said that he would now be expected to live much longer. There was also a woman in this video who said that laughter was the best medicine, who made fun of stress and worries, and whose message was not to take life too seriously.

Another tape pointed out that atherosclerosis starts early, in the teenage years, especially if genetic factors are present. It emphasized that even children should follow a heart-healthy diet and should control their weight.

My cardiologist told me that after my discharge I should take daily walks, but I was not to return to work for six weeks.

That was a problem for me. I am a research packaging engineer for a large semiconductor company, and we were in the process of developing a new method of packaging semiconductors that would result in a 40 percent reduction in the size and weight of the package. I am one of the key persons involved in this development, so even though I did not go into the office,

I kept in touch by e-mail during the entire six weeks, working two or three hours a day from home to make sure my project was going forward.

I did follow my cardiologist's other instruction and walked every day, initially for fifteen to twenty minutes. I gradually increased the time and tempo, until I walked for thirty to forty minutes at a fast pace. (Today I walk even faster.)

During this period I tried to learn as much as I could about heart attack from the Internet. I looked up the causes of atherosclerosis, and the significance of HDL and LDL cholesterol. I was very disappointed at the meager information that was available.

Apparently a number of risk factors for heart attack interact, but after looking at the various possibilities, I decided the only risk factor I had at the time of my heart attack was that total cholesterol/HDL ratio of 5. I did not really have a family history; my 86-year-old mother began to develop angina when she was about 80, which does not seem abnormal to me. I find my work relaxing and enjoyable, though sometimes the bureaucracy gets frustrating. Having been in both management and research in Puerto Rico (I'm a Puerto Rican American), I eventually decided to concentrate on the latter, which I enjoy very much.

While still in the hospital, one of the nurses provided me with a great deal of information about rehabilitation. (In fact, we heart attack patients were encouraged to walk the corridors of the hospital for exercise as early as possible.) She suggested I take part in cardiac rehabilitation, and after visiting a local program and watching the participants, I joined it as soon as my cardiologist cleared me to return to work.

Since I still work full time, I go to the evening classes. Just before leaving my office at 5:00 p.m., I often kid about having to go to my cardiac rehabilitation program. Although I do so in jest, I realize that it gives me a good excuse to leave the office instead of lingering over an unresolved problem. This was one advantage of the evening classes, but I would have looked forward to the classes in any case.

To me, the most important benefit of the cardiac rehabilitation program is that it is very structured, particularly with regard to the warm-up and cool-down procedures. I feel comfortable with structure. Then, too, all the participants and nurses are extremely friendly and pleasant to be around.

Having been a participant in a rehabilitation program for such a short time, I have only had a chance to attend two of the forums. One, about diet, was especially helpful.

The person who runs these forums asked for suggestions for future events and, as a newcomer, I find that I do have thoughts. I would be interested in a high-level technical discussion of the workings of the drugs I take, and how to handle the side effects. For example, the combination of statin drugs and niacin can damage the liver, although this is unlikely. I also wonder whether diet, exercise, and medication can actually reverse, not simply halt, atherosclerosis. If so, would it be possible for me to cut back on medication, so as to reduce the possibility of side effects?

What I Have Learned

After all that has happened, here is what I have learned:

- That in this new millennium, a cardiologist will usually take an angiogram within an hour of admission to the hospital, followed by either an angioplasty and stent (as in my case) or, if necessary, referral to a surgeon for bypass surgery. (The current goal is to perform angioplasty within two hours of presentation of symptoms.)
- That total cholesterol/HDL ratio should be 3 or less. In my case it was 5, which was my only risk factor for a heart attack.
- That heart patients are generally up and walking shortly after a heart attack and continue walking and exercising as soon as they are discharged.

- That patients are usually discharged from the hospital shortly after a heart attack, in my case after only three days.
- That if patients want to join a cardiac rehabilitation program, they can do so within a relatively short period after their heart attack.

CHAPTER 3

Doing It My Way

Hans Forsell

On February 21, 2000, I woke up at 6:00 a.m. feeling pressure at the center of my chest. I assumed the pressure would go away, so I went ahead with my daily routine—shower, coffee—after which I got ready for work.

As I drove to the office, the feeling of pressure in my chest increased, and I became more and more uncomfortable. I decided I needed to have it checked out; even though I was only 47, I began to wonder if I was having a heart attack.

I turned around and drove to the emergency room of the community hospital located just a block from my home, in the city on the east coast where I live. This hospital has an excellent reputation, especially for the treatment of heart disease.

I parked my car and walked around to the emergency room, where I told the receptionist I thought I might be having a heart attack.

The staff immediately gave me oxygen, attached some kind of device that measured the oxygen content of my blood, as well as a heart monitor with an electrocardiogram, which showed what the doctor called "marked S-T elevation." Yes, I was indeed having a heart attack. My blood pressure was very high, 225/100. I was told that I looked pale, and I was sweating profusely.

The staff drew blood to test for heart enzymes; later, they

would do this every eight hours to determine whether those enzyme levels were coming down.

At about 7:30 that morning, I called my wife, a cardiac nurse, who was still at home. She spoke to the nurse and to the emergency room physician on the phone. Initially, the doctor tried to soft-pedal what had happened, but when my wife identified herself and her profession, he said: "Okay, your husband has had an inferolateral myocardial infarct. We could treat him with clotbuster drugs, but we think an immediate angioplasty is a better bet."

Her response was, "Well, fine," and she asked the identity of the interventional cardiologist on call that day. She happened to know the person, which was very comforting.

My wife arrived at 7:50, just as I was being wheeled into the angio room. Less than two hours after the first symptoms, the cardiologist took a coronary angiogram. It showed a complete blockage of the left anterior descending artery, below the diagonal artery. The exact location was very fortunate, in that a smaller portion of my heart muscle would be affected.

The cardiologist performed an immediate angioplasty, which opened up the blocked artery. There was a slightly abnormal movement in a small part of the wall of my heart, indicating some injury to the heart muscle itself; this has now reverted to normal, because the cardiologist was so quick to open the blocked artery. Unfortunately, the cardiologist was unable to place a stent within the artery, because the artery itself was too small.

Following the procedure, the feeling of pressure in my chest immediately disappeared and the artery did not go into spasm, as sometimes happens. I still had S-T elevation on my electrocardiogram for a couple of days, which is a frequent occurrence in cases like mine.

I was kept flat on my back for six hours after the catheterization, to be sure that the artery in which the catheter had been inserted did not bleed. There were no complications, though, and the next morning I was allowed to get up and walk around.

After two days I was transferred from the coronary care unit to a general medical ward (they needed a bed, and I was in the best shape to move). On the third day after the procedure, I was discharged.

As my postoperative care commenced, I discovered that I had several risk factors for a heart attack, including smoking two packs of cigarettes a day, high blood pressure, stress, and a family history of coronary artery disease. (My father had had a heart attack in his sixties—three of his coronary arteries were diseased—together with recent complications that had caused me great stress. My 48-year-old brother developed type 2 diabetes at age 37, but has no evidence of heart disease.)

I was told to quit smoking. My doctors had had a great deal of difficulty controlling my blood pressure even before the heart attack. The stress was the result of my father's illness. He had been diagnosed with an abdominal aortic aneurysm two years earlier, but shortly before my own heart attack a number of other complications set in. After being advised, for example, not to have an operation, he got a second opinion and ultimately did have the operation. The aneurysm turned out to be huge. It actually burst on the operating table. In addition, my father, who had told his physician that he was not allergic to any antibiotics, had a severe anaphylactic reaction to one of the antibiotics he was given during surgery. These problems, along with others that developed postoperatively, were a source of great anxiety for the entire family, especially for me.

I had no additional risk factors for coronary artery disease: my weight was normal, as were my cholesterol, HDL and LDL, and triglyceride levels. But I was told to eat less fat and less red meat, to avoid caffeine, and to cut back on salt because of my high blood pressure.

My wife, as a nurse herself, was extremely disappointed in the information the hospital nurses gave me about cardiac rehabilitation—probably because I was discharged from a general medical ward instead of from the coronary unit. (The staff of a medical ward are less familiar with heart attack patients and are busy with unrelated matters.) This particular hospital has the best cardiac rehabilitation program in the area. My wife felt that one or two participants from the program should therefore speak to patients about the program and its benefits immediately after their heart attack, before discharge.

All I was told was that I would need cardiac rehabilitation, and that I would need to seek out a program myself. No one tried to enroll me in an existing program—to the dismay of my wife. I was told to walk fifteen minutes a day and gradually for longer, not to drive or engage in strenuous activity for six weeks, and not to return to work for six weeks.

When I was discharged, I was given prescriptions for Vasotec®, an ACE inhibitor that lowers blood pressure; Dyazide®, a diuretic that also lowers blood pressure; Toprol® for blood pressure control; and I was told to take one baby aspirin a day to help prevent blood clotting.

In the seven months since I left the hospital, I have reduced my smoking from two packs a day to one and am trying to decrease it still further. I have adhered faithfully to the recommended diet. But I also decided not to join a cardiac rehabilitation program, principally because of my cultural background.

My mother was of Scandinavian descent, and I grew up in Norway and Germany. That environment has always had a strong influence on me. Men from those cultures do not express their feelings, and they would find, as I did, the concepts of group therapy and cardiac rehabilitation to be strange and foreign. My joining any such group would have been totally out of character—I just could not do it.

Furthermore, I knew no one in any local cardiac rehabilitation program and would have felt uncomfortable. I believed that people in cardiac rehabilitation programs are usually a lot older than I am, and this was a problem. I was not offered any home-based program, in which I might have done rehabilitation on my own, with my progress constantly monitored.

(My wife feels that if someone from a rehab program, especially someone with a Scandinavian background, had visited me in the hospital, my reservations could have been addressed and I would have been more likely to join a program.)

At any rate, I now have my own walking program: I walk briskly for at least an hour a day, every day.

What I Have Learned

After all that has happened, here is what I have learned:

- That it is very important not to ignore the warning signs of a heart attack. A feeling of pressure in the center of the chest means that there is a problem—it will not go away, and it needs immediate attention.
- That once the diagnosis of heart attack is made, it is crucial to be treated as quickly as possible. If I had not had angioplasty within two hours of my first symptoms, my heart muscle could have been significantly more damaged. I have indeed been fortunate; since the surgery I have had no angina and no shortness of breath. Immediately after the heart attack I did tire more easily, but my stamina has improved dramatically.
- That it is possible to conduct your own cardiac rehabilitation. I should point out, though, that my wife feels that doing it on my own is harder, because I do not have the benefit of the encouragement of other members of the group. Also, cardiac rehabilitation programs frequently offer stress- and smoking-reduction programs, so it might thereby have been easier for me to stop smoking.
- That heart attack is serious. My own has given me pause and led me to reconsider my values and priorities.

CHAPTER 4

It Takes a Team

Max Kramer

August 20, 1988—a date I will not forget. On that day I joined a new team. I did not plan to become a participant, and I did not know at the time that the team would become a focus of my life. As I look back, I recognize that the team has had various members and that my own participation ranged from the initial passivity of being worked on in a hospital emergency room to a highly active role in understanding and managing my chronic cardiovascular disease. Many people have been part of my team since that fateful day; some played only fleeting roles, while others have held central and enduring positions. Let me describe some of the key players on my team and how they have contributed to lengthening my life and improving its quality.

It all began that Saturday morning as I was sitting at my computer working with a statistical package. The data analysis was going smoothly and I was getting some interesting results. I did not feel under any particular stress. I was looking forward to going to professional meetings on Monday morning, but since I was not scheduled to present this research at the meetings, there was no urgency to finish the analysis before I left. My family was in reasonably good shape, so I had no worries on that score.

Suddenly, just before noon, I felt very dizzy and began to perspire furiously. I did not feel any pain except for a low-level ache in my right arm and shoulder, which I attributed to muscle soreness. I started feeling weaker and weaker and dizzier and dizzier. My wife was in another part of the house engaged in a lengthy phone conversation with a colleague, and I did not want to interrupt her. So I thought I would just lie down until the spell passed. I had had an allergy shot earlier that morning, and my first thought was that I was having a reaction. In retrospect, my behavior was not very sensible; if it had been an allergic reaction, I should have moved quickly to get an adrenaline shot. But I guess I was not thinking too clearly at the time.

Lying down did not seem to help. The dizziness got worse and the weakness increased. After about ten minutes, I made what turned out to be the first move to involve others: I called out to my wife, who at that moment became a key member of my team (as she is today). I staggered to the kitchen where she was on the phone and told her that I didn't feel well—the first of many understatements of the day. Seeing that I was a ghostly shade of gray, she abruptly ended her conversation and took charge. For the rest of that day I was a very passive player.

Although these events took place twelve years ago, I have clear memories of what happened and some of my reactions. My wife called the urgent care unit at the clinic to which we had belonged for thirty years, and they told her to bring me in right away. When we arrived, the waiting room was crowded, but the triage nurse took one look and immediately ushered me into one of the examining rooms. Virtually the only thing I remember about that examination is two doctors solemnly telling me that I was having a heart attack. To which I replied, "Thanks a lot." They called the paramedics to take me to a nearby hospital.

The paramedics arrived quickly, loaded me into their ambulance, and put me on oxygen. I appreciated their quick professional response to my emergency. They started an intravenous drip, and I remember thinking that it was just like a television show. Then we sat and waited what seemed an eternity, but was only about ten minutes. The difficulty was that the paramedics were unable to establish radio contact with the hospital emergency room; they were getting ready to take me to a more distant hospital, but I urged them to take me to the medical center that was only five minutes away. This center had an international reputation for cardiac surgery; I was familiar with the hospital from a previous illness, and clinic physicians were members of the attending staff. Finally the paramedics made contact and we were off to the next stage in the day's drama.

Less than forty-five minutes from my wife's call to urgent care, I was wheeled into the emergency room on a gurney and surrounded by what seemed like a cast of thousands. The cardiac team had doctors, nurses, technicians, attendants, and a few other people I could not identify. The paramedics had alerted them, so they had had time to organize before receiving me. The team moved quickly to examine me and to begin treatment. They already had an EKG strip that was transmitted from the ambulance, but someone took a blood sample and someone else hooked me up to a monitor that continuously measured my vital signs. I remember a young woman resident asking the physician in charge of the team if she could give me a tranquilizer, since "the patient seems quite anxious." That was the second understatement of the day.

When the tranquilizer took effect, a strange transformation took place. I became a detached observer of what was happening, rather the victim of the events. I was no longer anxious, but instead was keenly interested in what was going on around me. Before the tranquilizer, I worried about how my wife was handling the shock; I hadn't seen her since urgent care. After the tranquilizer, that and my other concerns seemed to vanish and I became the neutral observer of an intellectual problem-solving exercise in which I was only incidentally involved.

In the emergency room, I was given a clotbusting drug. Since it was still experimental, I was asked to sign a document giving my informed consent. I remember thinking that this was a helluva time for paperwork; in retrospect, I'm not sure if I was in any condition to give informed consent—or if I could even have understood the implications of what I was being told. Never-

theless, I signed, probably with the unvoiced hope that the
team knew what they were doing. It probably helped that I
was slightly acquainted with the lead doctor, having met him
socially on a few occasions. Future events demonstrated that
confidence in this physician was well placed. He would play an
important part in decisions three years down the road.

The next thing I remember is seeing my arteries on a TV
monitor. The team took an angiogram and I watched as the clot
in my artery dissolved. When it disappeared, a cheer went up
from everyone in the room. I myself was thrilled at the sight and
later, as the head of the team performed a balloon angioplasty, I
was fascinated to watch the skillful movement of the thin wires
in my artery. Throughout all the procedures carried out that
afternoon, procedures that lasted more than four hours, I was
impressed by the skill, calmness, and humanity of all the people
working on me. Most outstanding was the way they functioned
as a team; each member knew his or her job; there was an obvious hierarchy, and feedback went both up and down the chain
of command. Ever the sociologist, I couldn't resist commenting.
I told the young woman resident that I did research on the pro-
ductivity of teams, and I thought this team was very effective.
Both she and the team leader found my comment amusing!

After the angioplasty an attendant wheeled me to the intensive care unit (ICU). We met my wife in the corridor and she accompanied us in the elevator. She told me she had spoken with
the head of the cardiac team, and he had reassured her that I
had a good chance to survive. (I found out years later that he
told her some other things that were not so favorable.) My wife
told me that she had called one of my colleagues, who immediately came to the hospital and sat with her during the time the
team was working on me. We were both very grateful to him,
and this was the real beginning of my appreciation of the importance of social support for the patient and the patient's immediate family.

That evening, various doctors and nurses told us that the
next twenty-four or forty-eight or seventy-two hours were criti-

cal. Probably all were correct, but the different stories were not as reassuring as they were meant to be. During the first few hours in the ICU, getting fed was my chief concern; in light of all that had happened since noon—a major heart attack, diagnosis at urgent care, treatment in the emergency room, and angioplasty—it amazes me that something so mundane could become so important to me. By the time I was ready to eat, the patient kitchen had closed, so someone went to the hospital cafeteria and brought me back a sandwich. At that moment, this anonymous member of my team was as much of a hero to me as those who had saved my life.

My wife stayed with me for several hours, during which I chatted animatedly about the angioplasty and what had happened during the time she had been outside waiting. Several times a nurse came in to try and shut me down. I was supposed to be lying quietly to avoid any bleeding from the angioplasty punctures in my groin. Since the team had given me anticlotting agents to prevent further cardiovascular attacks, it was difficult for the puncture wounds to heal even though they were small. For me, however, lying quietly is not easy unless I am asleep. Besides, it was important to talk, to share my experiences and feelings, and to vent some of my emotions. Both of us were in the middle of an episode that we had shared only partially. Recounting the events of the day and our reactions to them had great significance as a bonding act. The availability of someone to whom you can let it all out is critical to the therapeutic process.

During that day and evening I ran the gamut of emotions. While my wife was with me, I was on a high, a combination of the Valium® and elation at still being alive. After she left, reality began to press in on me. I was a very sick man who might not survive the night or the next day or the next week. I was afraid—afraid of the future, afraid of moving too suddenly and triggering a catastrophic event, afraid of dying, and afraid of living a constricted life. For the first time that day I was depressed. The ICU nurses spotted my problem and, although they tried to keep me quiet, they chatted with me at every opportunity in an effort to raise my lagging spirits. And it worked, although I paid a small price. Not lying as still as I should have led to more bleeding from my punctures. Pressure was needed in order to stop the bleeding. There I was lying in a hospital bed with a nurse pressing her hand on my groin for several hours; I realized that I wasn't dead yet when I recognized that she was both young and attractive.

Eventually the bleeding stopped and I fell asleep. It was about one in the morning, a little more than twelve hours after the episode had begun. While I wasn't sure that I would ever wake from this sleep, I was confident that many people on my team were watching out for me. The monitoring devices beeped steadily, giving me confidence that should something go wrong, a member of the cardiac care team would come to my aid immediately.

I never met all of the people on my team during this critical period, since some worked for me while I was asleep. The ones I did meet were not only calm and efficient but cheerful and upbeat. They all helped restore my confidence that I was going to make it. Building this confidence was a slow process, however, and it was several weeks before I was able to go to sleep without considering whether or not I would wake up the next morning.

The day after the surgery, my wife arrived shortly after breakfast, and my daughter came in from Arizona later in the day. My son was on vacation and not reachable. By this time, many of my friends and colleagues knew that I was in the hospital and wanted to visit me. Colleagues and students who were leaving the next day for the professional meeting that I would now miss wished to see me before they went. This created some problems. First of all, hospital policy allowed only family members to visit patients in the cardiac unit; second, space was extremely tight in the unit, so that there was barely room for two people to visit at one time; third, the unit was so crowded that conversations could easily be disturbing to the other patients. The nursing staff worried about my becoming unduly excited. My wife, however, knew that seeing my friends and students would be a tonic, so she negotiated with the nurses. They agreed to let me have two visitors at a time if those visitors would limit their stay to ten minutes each.

Late Sunday morning the parade began. I chatted spiritedly for most of the day; I had to tell every visitor all the details. Several times a nurse would try to enforce the negotiated rules, or warn that I needed a rest, or just try to quiet our noisy conversation. One nurse even threatened to stop the visitations, but we went right on. I don't know if all this activity disturbed any of the other patients or set back their recovery, but the visits were certainly a boon to me.

I would have talked nonstop, but my wife acted as a traffic cop, shuttling people in and out and making sure that I had some rest periods. In addition, every time someone needed to do a procedure on me, I was forced to keep quiet for a while. Then there were some lulls in the stream of visitors, during which I spent relatively quiet time with my wife and daughter; after all, they had heard my story more than once. Before the day was over, I had had more than two dozen visitors. Even though I had always understood the importance of relationships in my life, this was my first insight into their importance to the recovery process.

Three other significant occurrences during my hospital stay started putting my rehabilitation team in place. On Monday I met the cardiologist whom my primary care physician had selected for me. From our first meeting, he took the time to give me full explanations and to answer my questions as completely as he could. I've always appreciated his dealing with me as a full partner in my medical care.

The second significant event was my introduction to cardiac rehabilitation. The cardiac nurses who were responsible for patient education provided my wife and me with information about what to do on leaving the hospital, on the importance of proper diet and regular exercise, and on how to live with cardiovascular disease. Their most dramatic impact on my life, however, was their description of a local Phase III cardiac rehabilitation program. Phase III begins after one fully recovers from a myocardial infarction (MI) or from cardiac surgery and can last for the rest of one's life. I knew about exercise, although I had led a very sedentary life and believed that exercise could kill you! My wife, who was very knowledgeable about diet, had persuaded me to start eating less fat about a year before my MI. But the concept of Phase III rehabilitation was totally new to both of us and we did not grasp its full import until I had participated in the program for quite some time. These nurses did convince me that exercise was crucial, and I agreed to look into the rehab program as a way to exercise regularly. I knew that without a scheduled commitment, I would not have the discipline to exercise sufficiently.

The third happening was that I found a friend with whom I could share my illness, knowing that it was similar to his own. When I left the cardiac unit, I moved into a semiprivate room; a man approximately my age was in the other bed; he had had an MI the day before I did. We discovered a network of mutual friends when one of his visitors turned out to be a friend of mine as well. Our professions were somewhat related and we had many similar interests and prejudices. About six weeks after his hospital stay, he too joined the cardiac rehabilitation program, and we have served as sympathetic ears and travel consultants for each other ever since. We ride our stationary bikes at class and try to solve the world's problems.

Having an MI is an educational process that continues beyond the six weeks of recuperation. I quickly learned that healthy friends really do not want to hear about one's symptoms, or one's treatments, or one's dietary concerns; such conversation either bores them or raises their anxieties. Sharing with fellow sufferers, however, helps air feelings and problems and is a learning experience for both teller and listener. Not only do we gain knowledge through these discussions, but we experience emotional learning as well. Being part of a group that is dealing with a set of common health problems has contributed enormously to my rehabilitation.

During my hospital stay and for the six weeks of recuperation at home, I was a fairly passive member of my rehabilitation team. I saw my cardiologist several times and followed his directions. I watched my diet and took several short walks every day. I did not focus actively on my disease; I wanted to get it behind me and return to my work. Most of the time my mood was fairly upbeat, but I was sufficiently fearful that I had no inclination to extend myself physically or mentally. Toward the end of the six weeks, I began to work a few hours a day and did something I had never done before: I walked to and from my office and felt a sense of accomplishment that I could cover the mile back and forth without being at all tired. This small achievement gave me confidence enough to take the next step in my rehabilitation.

Joining the cardiac rehab program was the beginning of my taking responsibility for the management of my own disease. When my wife and I went for an interview with the director of the program, we did not know what to expect. I knew the program offered exercise classes supervised by cardiac nurses, but I had no idea of the range of additional benefits it provided. In the course of that interview I began to learn. The first lesson was that the program regarded rehabilitation as a lifetime affair. It was heartening to be told that some participants had been with the program since its founding nearly eighteen years earlier.

As if she were reading my mind, the director assured me that exercise would reduce rather than increase my risk. We also discussed other risk factors and how to control them. I thought I was fairly sophisticated, for a lay person, about factors like smoking and cholesterol, but I quickly discovered the shortcomings of my understanding. I began to appreciate just how crucial health information is to improving one's chances of survival and/or enhancing the quality of life. The program nurses became a major source of authoritative information and, more important, validators of intelligence obtained from other sources. This function is critical in a world where the media bombard us with health information and new health sites appear every day on the Internet.

When I joined the cardiac rehabilitation program, I added a number of extremely valuable members to my team. The program nurses not only supervised the members' exercise, but monitored our health status, our medications, and any side effects they might produce; provided a rationale for what our cardiologists or primary care physicians prescribed; and gave us the support and psychological impetus to maintain a heart-healthy regime. A major theme of the program is that the patient needs to take responsibility for his or her own health, but there is also the recognition that an individual cannot do it alone.

It took me some time to integrate myself into the cardiac rehab program. In the beginning, I was fearful of the exercises; I hesitated to ask questions of the nurses; I was reluctant to discuss my experiences with fellow participants. Never well coordinated, I was afraid to look foolish doing the warm-up and stretching exercises. Once, the exercise leader corrected me in one of the stretches and I was mortified. Two factors helped draw me into full participation: the warmth and solicitousness of the staff, and the presence of my hospital roommate, whose gregariousness was contagious.

In my growth as a full participant in the program, I became aware of the critical importance of social and psychological support. Although I am very close to my wife and children, I needed support from people who understood the experience of living with the silent time bomb of cardiovascular disease. At almost every exercise class, one of the nurses would draw me out, making me express my concerns and offering strategies to handle them. With the aid of my hospital roommate and a few other members whom I had known outside the program, I became friendly with many other participants, who became part of my support team.

My first three years in the rehab program were relatively uneventful. To my surprise, I came to enjoy the exercise and admitted that I felt better after a workout. I benefited from the nutritional information the program disseminated, and from an eight-session stress management course the program provided. I shared cardiac experiences with many individuals. I developed a deep appreciation for the program director, the assistant director, the nurses, and the exercise leaders. The time I spent in rehab class became increasingly meaningful to me; when I was out of town on business or on vacation, I really missed the class even when I was able to exercise elsewhere. Intellectually, socially, and emotionally, I was part of a caring community.

About three years after my MI, I discovered just how important my cardiologist is to my continued survival. I have a bundle branch blockage, thus ordinary stress tests are not informative; furthermore, when I had my attack, I did not suffer any pain. Since the stress test was not useful and since I did not have the usual warning sign of impeding cardiac difficulties—angina —my doctor decided that I needed an annual cardiac scan to monitor my heart.

A nuclear medicine physician reads the scan and reports to the cardiologist, who frequently studies the scan as well. My first two scans showed that my heart had sustained damage in the original attack, but had been relatively stable since. After my third annual scan, the nuclear medicine physician reported that the situation was pretty much the same as the previous year. In looking at the pictures, however, my cardiologist did not like what he saw. Returning several times to the current scan and comparing it with past scans, he recommended that I have an angiogram.

The angiogram confirmed my cardiologist's uneasiness. He strongly advised me to have bypass surgery. He told me that it was not an emergency and that he hated to propose a drastic procedure for someone not showing any symptoms. He felt, however, that I was running a very high risk of a fatal episode if I did not have the surgery within the next year. He counseled me to get a second opinion before deciding.

I consulted the physician who headed the cardiac team that had treated my original MI, the head of the catheterization lab at the medical center. Not only did he concur with my cardiologist's recommendation, but he quickly convinced me by showing me the videotape taken during my angiogram. A significant portion of my heart was not pumping; either the muscle was dead or it was hibernating because of insufficient blood flow. If part of the muscle were merely hibernating, bypass surgery would correct the condition; in terms of survival and enhancing the quality of life, it was certainly worth the gamble.

I was intensely fearful of any kind of surgery and of the possible postsurgical pain, but I felt I had no choice. My intention was to schedule the surgery as soon as possible rather than fret over it for months. I arranged for an appointment with a highly recommended cardiac surgeon, and my wife and I went see him. Although I have no complaint about his work, that appointment and a brief hospital visit the night before the surgery were the only times I saw the surgeon. And I remember very little about either meeting. Whether my relative amnesia is due to my anxiety at the time or to the lack of anything memorable about the conversations, I cannot say. I do recall telling him that I had read that the mortality rate for this surgery was 1–2 percent and then asking what his rate was. Without bragging, he said that his rate was quite a bit better. While his comment should have reassured me, my statistical training apparently defeated me; while the odds were certainly in my favor, I knew that I could be the one failure in a million.

During this interlude the cardiac rehab program was a tremendous source of support. The nurses and other class members spent a great deal of time helping me cope with my fears. Nearly half of my exercise class had had the surgery and many eagerly shared their experiences with me. One person who was in the program with his wife gave me a detailed account of how easily I would get through the surgery and the recuperation period. It was only later that I discovered that *he* had not had the surgery but was giving me the benefit of his wife's experience. My fellow participants tried to give me clear ideas of what to expect and to virtually guarantee that I would come out of the surgery feeling much better than when I went in. Since I was symptom free and felt pretty well, I did not know how to react to these assurances. Still, the compassionate concern helped me through a rough period.

I went into the hospital on a Sunday, the day before the surgery. My wife, my son, and his girlfriend accompanied me. The day went smoothly and we even managed to be lighthearted—until we saw a video about the surgery and the postsurgical recovery. The video was intended to be informative about what to expect, and I suppose it accomplished its purpose. But seeing a patient with all sorts of tubes emerging certainly scared the wits out of us.

That night, after my visitors left, I had separate visits from the surgeon and the anesthesiologist. The anesthesiologist gave me a detailed description of what she planned for me and what my likely reactions would be. The surgeon's visit was very brief and I wasn't quite sure of its purpose. It was the last time I ever saw him; I assume that he was in the operating room, and he undoubtedly did a fine job or I wouldn't be writing about it now.

Despite my anxiety, I managed to get a decent night's sleep, and I think it was unaided. I was awakened very early Monday morning for the prep work. My wife was with me when they brought the gurney to take me to the operating room, and she helped keep me relatively calm. I recall the nurse starting an IV, and the next thing I knew it was Wednesday afternoon. I had been out for more than forty-eight hours. While I was spared the anxiety of that Monday and Tuesday, my wife bore the full brunt. Fortunately, my son and his friend stayed with her during the six hours I was in surgery, and some of our friends stopped by at the waiting room to give their support.

By the time I woke up on Wednesday, the surgical residents had removed all the pipes and tubes from my chest. I did not feel any pain. I remember that I was very hungry and had some soreness in my chest, but I was elated because I was still alive. The surgery had gone smoothly and the outcome was successful; the part of my heart that had not been pumping started up again, indicating that it actually had been in hibernation.

This hospital stay once again brought home to me the importance of my network of relationships. On Thursday morning I moved out of intensive care, and then began a deluge of visitors. I was in no shape to entertain, but these calls provided a boost for my recovery and reassurance that what I was experiencing was typical. The director of the cardiac rehab program, several of the nurses, and one of the exercise leaders came to see me and their visits raised my spirits. On Friday I was acting pretty strangely, and two of the rehab nurses independently assured my wife that I would get over this and be back to my normal self in a short time. (I did and I was.) Several participants in the rehab program also came to see me and gave me good advice to aid my recuperation. Of course, family, friends, and professional colleagues visited, so my days were pretty full. So many people dropped in that one of the hospital staff asked me if I were running for office.

Two events marred my recovery, and I mention them because to me they indicate flaws in the system that need to be dealt with. I picked up a thrush infection that made my throat and mouth very sore and interfered with eating. No one understood how much discomfort I suffered, so the residents and nurses declined to give me anything to clear it up until I was ready to leave the hospital. The chief resident who saw me twice a day was helpful on everything else, but did not appreciate how much discomfort I suffered from this infection.

The other event was partly my own fault. The day before my surgery I was asked to participate in a study dealing with recovery from bypass surgery. I strongly believe in the value of research, and before my surgery I felt well, so I volunteered. I should have told the investigator to see me after the surgery— when, if I felt up to it, I would participate in her study. Since I had agreed to take part, she appeared on Friday, my worst day, to take me for one and a half hours of scans. I found these scans quite painful, and I tried several times to persuade the researcher to stop and return me to my room. But she would not let go; she continued until she finished, oblivious to my severe distress. Since research subjects were hard to find, apparently she was not going to lose one! If I was crazy and uncomfortable before this experience, I was a physical and emotional wreck after it. Fortunately, my bizarre state did not last very long, and on Sunday I went home to begin five more weeks of convalescence.

For the first two weeks at home, I could not do much but walk and sleep. I could not concentrate enough to read even a novel. Of course, I could not go to rehab class, but the program came to me. Those who had visited me in the hospital, as well as many others, came again during those two weeks, and I am sure they speeded my psychological recovery. Physically, I was able to do a little more each day. I started taking four quarter-mile walks a day, each followed by a nap. By the time I was cleared to return to exercise class, I was taking one two-mile walk a day and not napping at all.

Initially, I saw my cardiologist once a week and he was very encouraging. He ordered another cardiac scan, and it confirmed that the hibernating part of my heart was once again pumping. After the fourth week, he allowed me to go back to work full time and to drive a car. Other than cautioning me not to overdo and to continue to take my medications, he placed no restrictions on my activities. One month later, less than ten weeks after my surgery, I climbed the approximately 150 steps to the top of Mont-Saint-Michel in France without even stopping to catch my breath.

The next six years were relatively uneventful. I continued my participation in the rehab program, attending exercise class three times a week, listening to the educational lectures the program sponsored, and consulting with the nurses when questions arose about medications, symptoms, and media health reports. I was so grateful for all the support I had received that I started to do my share of visiting other members who were hospitalized. I saw my cardiologist three or four times a year; by this time, he had become my primary care physician, so some of the consultations were unrelated to my cardiac problems.

In the winter of 1998 I came down with a severe respiratory infection. This time the usual remedies did not work, so after ten days I called my doctor for an antibiotic prescription. He gave me the prescription, but insisted that I get an X ray of my lungs. He called the next day to tell me that the X ray showed fluid in my lungs, a symptom of congestive heart failure; he immediately put me on a diuretic and indicated that he wanted me to continue taking it even after I was over the current episode. At my next office visit about two weeks later, the doctor discussed changing my regime. He told me that the best treatment for congestive heart failure involved a relatively new beta-blocker plus a diuretic. He had examined the results of an echocardiogram and felt that this was the direction to take. I had known that I had a damaged heart, but now I learned that it was becoming less efficient.

My cardiologist did not dwell on the test results but focused on the incident of water retention. Despite the fact that beta-blockers are contraindicated for patients with asthma (and I had infrequent, mild asthma), he was determined to go ahead with a regime involving carvedilol and a diuretic. Thus began a long period of acclimating me to a new medication.

Carvedilol is a drug that one cannot begin or end abruptly. The starting dosage is 3.125 milligrams twice a day, with the dosage doubling approximately every two weeks until the maximum of 25 milligrams twice a day is reached. The first level did not create any problems, but the 6.25 level was another story. I started wheezing and coughing every day and felt fatigued much of the time. I had occasional dizziness and often felt light-headed. I was sufficiently distressed by these side effects that I wanted to abandon the regime. Here once again the nurses of the cardiac rehab program were instrumental in persuading me to continue with carvedilol.

When I first started taking the drug, one of the nurses with some expertise in this area reinforced everything that my cardiologist had told me. She even brought me photocopies of research articles reporting large-scale studies evaluating the effectiveness of carvedilol, including one study that showed dramatic improvements in the prognosis for patients with mild heart failure. When I was quite discouraged by the symptoms I was experiencing, this nurse and the program director both urged me to continue. They assured me that the symptoms would disappear, or at least moderate, and argued that even if the side effects continued, they were a small price to pay for the long-term benefits. Had I been on my own, I probably would have told my doctor that I wanted to stop the medication. Knowing that I would have to face the nurses, however, convinced me not to "chicken out."

My cardiologist and the nurses were right. Although it took me more than four months to reach maximum dosage, the side effects gradually lessened in both frequency and severity. Today I am largely free of them. I have become a booster for the drug and have tried to give the benefit of my experience to others in the rehab program who have started on carvedilol.

I hope my story shows that I am active player on my own team and am taking major responsibility for managing my rehabilitation.

What I Have Learned

After all that has happened, here is what I have learned:

- That rehabilitation is a lifetime affair.
- That I am in control, but I have a lot of backup, ready to intervene if necessary.
- That I can obtain reliable information.
- That I have access to authoritative evaluators of health information.
- That there are people with whom I can share my illness-

related experiences and my reactions to those
experiences.
- That I can help myself and others cope with our shared
disease.

I am absolutely convinced that working with my team has
prolonged my life and increased its quality. One cannot expect
any one individual to perform all the diverse functions of lifetime cardiac rehabilitation—not the patient, not the patient's
spouse, not the physician, not a rehab nurse, and not a fellow
patient. Together, as a team, all these people contribute in crucial ways to a person's education, nutrition, physical activity,
and psychological and social well-being—and *that* constitutes
a comprehensive cardiac rehabilitation program.

CHAPTER 5

Reversing Angina

Helen L'Amoreaux

The evening of August 12, 1994, is one I will never forget.

We were on vacation in our summer cabin, which overlooked a magnificent unpolluted lake in the East, very close to the Canadian border. On the previous day, my 83-year-old husband, George, (I was then 75) had mused out loud how wonderful it was that we were in excellent health. And we were looking forward to celebrating the birthdays, on the twelfth, of our granddaughter and daughter-in-law.

On August 12 our son was driving his Volvo, which at the time had the highest safety rating of any car. He was driving 25 miles an hour (40 km/hr) in the right lane, the slow lane, through a small town about 30 miles (48 km) from our cabin. George was in the right front seat; I was in the left rear seat, next to my 16-year-old granddaughter and her mother, the birthday girls. We were all wearing seat belts.

All of a sudden a pickup truck came careening erratically toward us at about 50 miles an hour (80 km/hr) from the opposite right lane, across two lines of traffic and the left-turn lane on the opposite side, all the way to where we were, crossing two additional lanes on our side.

Our son had about six seconds to act. On his right, crowds of pedestrians lined the sidewalk, for it was a warm summer day.

On his left, a car was traveling beside us in the next lane. He had no other options; he braked, suddenly and hard.

George yelled, "What the . . ." The pickup struck the right front side of the Volvo; a deafening sound of steel crushing steel was followed by a brilliant flash of light. The truck rolled over. An eerie silence followed.

I immediately felt a terrific pain in my chest and belly and could not keep myself from moaning. My 16-year-old granddaughter asked, "Grandma, did I buckle your seat belt too tightly? Are you all right?" Trying to calm her, I gasped as confidently as I could, "No, I'm not all right, but I know I will be."

Poor George was also in a bad way: the truck had pushed the Volvo's engine into the passenger area, pinning his legs against his seat. (The Volvo is designed to behave this way in a crash. The idea is that in a head-on collision the engine moves backward and down, rather than backward and up—into a passenger's body.) George tried to unbuckle his seat belt, but he could not. His left arm was paralyzed.

At that moment, someone tapped on George's window. My son reached across and rolled the window down. A young woman stuck her head into the car and said, very quietly and gently: "I'm a registered nurse. Listen to my instructions. If you are injured, don't move." She opened George's door and freed his seat from the engine, which had impaled his legs. Noticing that he could not move his left arm, she realized immediately that he might have broken his neck. She carefully took hold of his head and kept it immobile for twenty minutes, while waiting for the ambulance to arrive.

Two ambulances and several police cars appeared. The paramedics thought I had life-threatening internal injuries and rushed me to a trauma center three miles away. They considered George's condition less immediately serious, and took him to a nearby general hospital. Fortunately, our grandchildren were uninjured, our son had a broken foot, and his wife's ribs were broken; my husband and I received the only serious injuries.

In the meantime, the police discovered that the truck driver was a young woman whose driver's license had been suspended because of substance abuse, and who had no insurance. Her blood alcohol concentration was unbelievable, almost twice the legal limit in California. Her male companion was also intoxicated. The driver eventually spent a year in prison for her crime.

Shortly after I arrived at the trauma center, the surgeon performed an exploratory laparotomy on me, which means simply that he opened my belly and looked around to see what the problems were. And he did discover some genuine, life-threatening injuries: my spleen was ruptured and bleeding, so he removed it; one area of my liver was lacerated, but he repaired it; and he reduced multiple rib fractures. X rays also revealed a compression fracture of my spine, about which he could do nothing.

When the surgeon saw me in the intensive care unit afterward, he told me quite candidly that he had been concerned that I might not survive, because of my age and because of the extent and type of my injuries. "But," he said, "when I examined you, I saw that your physical condition was unbelievably good." He asked me how I had kept myself in such great shape. "Because," I replied, "I have belonged to a cardiac rehabilitation program for the last twenty years."

"Yes, that's it!" he said.

Thus a cardiac rehabilitation program had saved my life for a second time. I will tell you shortly how it had reversed my coronary artery disease and saved my life the first time.

When George was taken to the general hospital, an X ray was taken of his neck while he was still on a stretcher in the ambulance. A young physician, age no more than 30, announced, "Son, you have a broken neck!" A bemused George was taken immediately to the trauma center where I was.

A terrific team, a neurosurgeon and his nurse wife, operated on George's neck. (He was the only neurosurgeon within 200 miles, it turned out.) He told George that his lower four cervical vertebrae had been fractured and displaced, and that he would have to graft bone to the vertebrae in order to stabilize them. So his wife harvested bone from George's right hip, while he worked on the neck itself.

The next day, the surgeon told George that it was a miracle he had survived. "If just one of your vertebrae had been displaced even a fraction of an inch more, your whole body would have been paralyzed from the neck down. It was sheer, blind luck that there was a nurse on the scene to immobilize your neck and prevent further damage."

It was also sheer, blind luck that George had come with me all those years to the exercises at the cardiac rehabilitation program. As a result, at age 83 he too was in wonderful physical condition and able to withstand both the initial impact and the subsequent surgery. "In fact," the surgeon went on, "you are so healthy that I think you will recover completely."

He was right. George did, and I did. We are both eternally grateful to the cardiac rehabilitation program for, in a very direct way, saving our lives.

Eleven days after our admission to the trauma center, the two of us were sent for three weeks to a nearby recovery center. Our apartment there had a bedroom, kitchen, and living room; our daughter came to stay with us and did all the cooking and the laundry.

After our discharge, we returned to our cabin on the beautiful lake, where a nurse from our insurance company visited at regular intervals to check on our progress. She was, she said, amazed at our fast recovery. "You are healing," she said, "at the rate of people fifty years younger." Soon we began the exercises we had learned at the cardiac rehabilitation program; I cooked, and George, with his neck immobilized in a halo, sawed wood for our fireplace. (In the end, the neurosurgeon removed the halo earlier than usual.)

Only one difficult problem lingered. I developed avian tuberculosis, the kind found usually in birds, not people. This odd disease has lingered for years, and I have had severe allergic reactions to the various medications used to treat it.

We had driven from California to our East Coast cabin, but our respective surgeons did not allow us to drive back until eight months had passed. That meant a winter in the woods, during which we cooked and chopped and sawed, injuries or no.

Why were we in a cardiac rehabilitation program at all? Before I answer that question, let me tell you more about us.

When I graduated from high school, it was clear that I could not afford to go to college, so for two years I worked in the advertising department of a magazine in Detroit. After I was admitted to Michigan State University, the magazine allowed me to work summers at the same monthly salary. In addition, in 1939, while I was still a student, I achieved two firsts: I was the first female hired by the *Detroit News* as an upstate reporter, and I was one of the first women accepted in a government pilot training course. I was granted a private pilot's license by the Civil Aeronautics Administration (later reorganized under the Federal Aviation Administration).

After graduation in 1941, I moved to Chicago, where George (a fellow pilot) and I decided to marry. Since we had no money, the wedding would be small; George's great-uncle, a Congregational minister, who had married his parents, agreed to marry us. He got sick on the day of our wedding, which was canceled. George was a commercial airline pilot and had to fly to Nashville immediately after what would have been the ceremony; I had been booked as a nonpaying passenger on the same flight, and we had looked forward to a honeymoon in Fort Worth, Texas.

Just as the flight was boarding, a high-ranking general arrived, demanding a seat. As the only nonpaying passenger, I was bumped. I was forced to stay illegally overnight in the crew room, but got a flight to Fort Worth the next day, whereupon we went directly to an Episcopal church and asked the bishop to marry us. "Impossible," he said; our banns would have to be published for three weeks before the marriage could take place. We told our best man about this and he said, "Let me deal with it." He went to the bishop and asked, "Which would you prefer, that they live in sin for three weeks or get married immediately?" The bishop chose the latter course and married us the next day, which was, of course, Halloween!

After World War II, George flew again for a commercial airline out of New York City, but at the end of 1962 he was transferred to San Francisco. He flew out of that city for the first time on New Year's Eve 1962.

After that initial flight, he felt ill. The nurse found that his blood pressure was very high; she called a physician, who confirmed the reading. The physician turned off the lights and took George through a thirty-minute schedule of relaxation exercises in the dark—but his blood pressure remained high. George was terrified; his mother had died of high blood pressure at the age of 69. We had three children in college and would have no money to pay tuition if he lost his job because of his blood pressure.

The doctor was reassuring. He put George through what was called a Master two-step test, the forerunner of today's treadmill examination, which George passed with flying colors. He was referred to a cardiologist, who successfully treated his high blood pressure with medications. The cardiologist discovered that George's blood pressure went up when he ate salty foods; the diagnosis was "essential salt-sensitive hypertension" and George was warned to restrict his salt intake.

This George did, but on two occasions he accidentally had too much salt. His body retained too much water, and he became breathless due to heart failure. Both times, we were vacationing in our cabin in the East. The first occasion was in 1988, when we were invited to a party at which there was an enormous buffet with acres of salty food. That food put George in a local hospital for three days, where he was put on diuretics to get rid of the excess water. The second episode occurred in 1990, when we dined in a restaurant that served very salty food. That time George was treated simply as an outpatient.

Apart from those two incidents, George has been extraordinarily fit despite his age (88 and counting). He is very active, walks upright with no difficulty, exercises vigorously, and is mentally as alert as ever. George retired in 1972. Knowing he would never be happy unless he was in the air, as a retirement gift I bought him a membership in a local flying club.

All was well with us until April of 1974, when one day I noticed a pain in my chest when I swam. At first I thought it might be some kind of cramp, but when the pain came back every time I swam, I realized it felt different; it was a constriction.

I went immediately to my internist, who did a resting electrocardiogram. It was normal. He told me I did not have coronary artery disease; after all, why would a fit 55-year-old woman with no family history of heart disease, a normal blood cholesterol, and a very normal electrocardiogram have coronary artery disease?

But I continued to have the constriction every time I swam.

One day George and I decided to take a flying-club plane to Lake Tahoe. I was the pilot on that occasion, but as soon as the plane, which was not pressurized, reached 4,000 feet (1,212 m), I felt the severe, constricting chest pain again, and we returned. The pain disappeared as we descended to sea level.

The next day I walked to the mailbox near our gate, and once again felt the pain—this time it was so severe that I had to rest on the way back to the house. By now the internist was taking my complaints more seriously, so he did a bicycle test, another forerunner of the modern treadmill exam. This time the result was positive for coronary artery disease. He repeated the test, and as soon as I developed the chest pain, he asked me to put a tablet of nitroglycerine (which relaxes the arteries) under my tongue. The pain immediately disappeared, and that, the internist said, confirmed the diagnosis: I had coronary artery disease.

The doctor sat me down and explained that there was now a brand-new test for this disease, the coronary angiogram. However, George's close friend, also a pilot, had developed angina and died on the table while undergoing this new procedure. The cause of death was some technical problem with the examination itself. I declined the procedure. (Of course, today the procedure is very safe, and no one would be concerned about associated risks.) The internist went on to say that he did have two recommendations. The first was that I take nitroglycerine whenever I developed chest pain; the second was that I join a cardiac rehabilitation program. To these suggestions I agreed.

George and I both joined the program. On the first day the two people in charge examined and tested us, then counseled us about diet and exercise.

All my life I had been a beef eater. But now, it appeared, I would have to reduce that consumption significantly, avoid butter, drink only skim milk, and eat only nonfat cheese. And I would be eating more whole grains and fresh fruits and vegetables.

The doctor in charge of the program prescribed a series of exercises for me, which were to begin with my jogging around a track for a minute, then walking for a minute, alternating for thirty minutes. I tried, but at first I could not do it.

But the doctor was right there on the track with me and said, "Okay, walk for one minute, then jog for only fifteen seconds, and alternate for thirty minutes." He and the nurses persisted, and slowly, bit by bit, I managed to increase the exercise until after about five years I was jogging a full thirty minutes every day with very little angina.

I also owe a lot to George, who encouraged me every step of the way. There were days when I did not feel like attending class; with great good cheer he would urge me to go. It was George who made sure that I followed the diet, and he encouraged me to swim, or water ski, or run, or hike, or climb mountains on days when there was no class.

Apart from the diet and exercise, the program had other benefits as well: the enormous encouragement and support we received from the nurses, and the mutual support we have had and continue to receive from others in our situation. We have also very much appreciated the health lectures given at the rehabilitation center.

In 1993 the program offered a new course, a modified Dean Ornish program. Once again, it was George who encouraged me to participate. Because of his persistence, we followed the Ornish diet exactly, becoming strict vegans and limiting our fat intake to 10 percent of daily calories. My own physician said that the Ornish diet was too strict for us and suggested that we modify it slightly by adding fish once or twice a week, and skinless chicken breast once every two weeks. This we did. George insisted that we follow this modified Ornish diet and eliminate beef from our diets entirely.

At about the same time I became entirely free of angina for the first time since it began. My treadmill test (by this time it had been invented) was normal. I was ecstatic; cardiac rehabilitation had actually *reversed* my coronary artery disease. I have had no angina since, and my treadmill tests since that wonderful moment have all been negative.

What I Have Learned

After all that has happened, here is what I have learned:

- That, amazingly, my angina disappeared when I combined exercise with an appropriate diet. After concentrating on exercise alone for a number of years, the pain I felt while exercising finally vanished. And my EKG became normal once I added the Ornish diet (with a little extra poultry and fish) to my exercise program.
- That my success in reversing the angina was also helped enormously by the fact that my husband endorsed and participated in all aspects of my rehabilitation—the diet, the exercise, the educational programs. It helped ease my own burden and kept me from thinking I was all alone with this problem. And it helped George to feel useful and to become an even more important part of my life than before.

CHAPTER 6

Preventive Medicine Works

Peter Jones

Most people do not associate heart attacks with African Americans. But I am an African American, and my elder brother died of a heart attack at age 47; I developed angina when I was 60.

In fact, African Americans have more heart attacks and strokes than Caucasians. High blood pressure is four times more common, and diabetes twice as common. One result is that heart attacks are more common in African American women than in Caucasian women, and tend to occur at an earlier age. For similar reasons, stroke and sudden death are more common in African Americans than in Caucasians—all of which suggests that African Americans need preventive medicine at least as much as anyone else.

All my close relatives died early: the elder brother I have mentioned, from a heart attack; another elder brother, from lymphoma; and my father, who was a heavy smoker, from lung cancer. My mother died from rheumatic heart valve disease, and most of my uncles and male cousins died early (one from a stroke, one in an automobile accident, and several from cancer). So all my life I have known that I would not live much beyond age 60. I have accepted this as calmly and as philosophically as I could.

I foolishly began to smoke when I was 17, although never

more than a pack or so a day; but when my father and so many close relatives died of cancer, I became very anxious about the effects of smoking on me and my three sons. So I quit when I was in my midthirties.

At age 25 I married a nurse. She insisted on a heart-healthy diet, which we followed year after year. We have always had a dog, which guaranteed that I would get at least some exercise, walking about a half a mile a day, seven days a week.

I was a senior manager at one of the largest companies in the United States. But being a manager apparently took its toll; so many died of heart attack at a young age that in 1985 the company decided to act. It offered a type A behavior modification program for all who wanted to participate, and, on our birthdays, all senior managers were required to have a medical checkup—on site, at a special medical facility the company paid for, and the best doctors money could buy.

On my sixtieth birthday, I had my first checkup. It was, as you can imagine, a crucial moment for me: I had never thought I would live much beyond it.

When the doctor asked if I had any symptoms, I replied that I had a lot of gas. He asked me to describe this "gas." I said that when I walked, I felt a pain, like a rubber band tightening on my chest. The doctor looked up and said that I had classic angina and that I needed to see a cardiologist immediately.

Not having an internist, I made an appointment directly with the cardiologist, who confirmed I was indeed having angina. On physical examination, I had high blood pressure; laboratory tests confirmed that my cholesterol levels were very high, while my HDL (good cholesterol) levels were very low. Thus, according to my cardiologist, my angina had at least three causes: high blood pressure, high cholesterol, and low HDL.

I took the news calmly. Right, I thought. Just as I predicted. Medical problems at age 60.

This new doctor did a coronary angiogram, which showed that I had some narrowing of the coronary arteries. He prescribed medicine to lower my blood pressure, niacin and colestid to lower cholesterol and raise HDL levels, and an aspirin a day to help prevent blood clot.

For about five years this strategy seemed to work.

But in 1990 I again developed angina, which required an angioplasty; and in 1992 the angina returned for a third time, and I had yet another angioplasty for a different artery. I felt totally relaxed and calm about both angioplasties; I tolerated them very well and experienced no discomfort whatsoever afterward.

So I am extremely grateful that my company had instituted a preventive medical program for its senior managers. If my coronary artery disease had not been diagnosed in the very early stages, who knows what might have happened! I might have had a heart attack at some point later on, I might have had to undergo coronary bypass surgery, or I might even have died of a heart attack. For obvious reasons, I am now a great believer in preventive medicine.

In that one of my brothers died young, of lymphoma, I was not too surprised when in 1986, just a year after my first coronary angiogram, the doctor discovered that I too had lymphoma. A radiation oncologist treated me with high doses of radiation and irradiated my thyroid gland, after which I was put on thyroid hormone tablets. All of this was to ensure that there would be enough thyroid hormone in my blood stream, to prevent elevating my blood cholesterol levels and worsening my coronary artery disease.

After my first angioplasty, the cardiologist referred me to a cardiac rehabilitation program. I attend the first classes of the day and, as I repeatedly comment to my wife, that class is the highlight of my day. Though I am now retired, it was the highlight even when I was still working, for each day started with a wholesome, invigorating session.

The two aspects of the program that have helped me the most are the physical exercise itself and the extraordinarily knowledgeable and attentive nursing staff. I have discovered that if I do not exercise first thing in the morning, I will not be exercising at all. And if I think I can only exercise at home, I may as well forget it; exercising by myself bores me. When I exercise in a group, there are always people to talk to, particularly on adjacent exercycles, and I have always found the conversation surprisingly stimulating.

Sometimes there are things I want to know about my medical and physical state that are too trivial (I always think) to ask my own doctor. For example, I have a bottle of medicine whose label says to take only on an empty stomach. What does "an empty stomach" mean? Do I wait one, two, three, or four hours after my last meal? What happens if I *don't* take the medicine on an empty stomach?

The nurses in the program have always been able to answer these kinds of questions and more, which not only spared me the embarrassment of asking my own doctor, but got me the information I needed and might otherwise have tried to live without. This sort of "embarrassment" can have serious consequences; fortunately, the wonderful nurses in our program help us avoid them.

Every day one of the nurses asks if I am having any problems. This routine is really helpful; sometimes a problem I thought was insignificant turns out to be very significant, in which case the nurse always suggests that I see my doctor immediately. In this way, problems dealt with early are kept from becoming serious. (If I had not attended rehab classes, I know that I would never have contacted my physician with what I considered insignificant problems.) In fact, my doctor claims that one of the biggest advantages of rehabilitation programs is that his patients are referred to him by the nurses when they are having early, treatable signs of disease, rather than when it may be too late.

Once I happened to frown slightly when I was exercising. Immediately a nurse rushed up and asked if I was feeling all right. This is just one example of how extraordinarily attentive our nurses can be, and it is the major reason I feel so strongly that it is the nurses, the incredible nurses, that make programs like this work.

There are other benefits to the program, of course, but for me, the two I have mentioned are the most important. I also have greatly enjoyed the health lectures, each of which has been excellent and helpful.

I know that for many people, the social aspects of this program are significant, but not for me. It is not that I have a problem with the people here; this is the only group to which I have ever belonged about which I can honestly say that there is not a single person I do not like. And I do like socializing with other folks on the exercycles. But I do not belong to this program to have a social life. I already have a very active social life outside the program, and after class I want to get home, shower, and get on with my day. I don't want to sit around drinking coffee and chatting idly.

So now, at the age of 75, I am deeply grateful to have lived fifteen years longer than I ever believed possible, and fourteen years longer than any of my relatives.

What I Have Learned

After all that has happened, here is what I have learned:

- That a significant factor in preventing my angina from progressing to a heart attack is that I worked for a farsighted company which had instituted a program of preventive medicine. The doctor there saw immediately that what I thought was gas pain was really angina. My experience has made me realize how important it is that everyone—particularly African Americans, in whom coronary artery disease is especially common—get regular medical checkups as they grow older.
- That once I knew what angina actually felt like, I was able to recognize it right away. When I experienced it twice

more, I got the appropriate medical attention. The angina was treated with angioplasty, which also helped prevent it from becoming a heart attack.

- That exercise and diet are other ingredients in preventing angina from becoming a heart attack and that, for me personally, a cardiac rehabilitation program is ideal. It encourages me to exercise and diet on a regular basis.

CHAPTER 7

Modern Cardiology, Cardiac Surgery, and My Angina

David Moses

Today is the day after my eighty-eighth birthday. I am celebrating, among other things, the fact that I am fit and healthy. How did this happen? Well, I think there are two reasons. First, my body has become a kind of showcase for the latest medical devices. Second, for the past twenty-five years I have belonged to a cardiac rehabilitation program.

Both my grandmothers lived into their eighties. One grandfather was killed in a railroad accident; the other died of "consumption" in his late fifties. My father lived into his nineties, my mother into her eighties. Heart trouble is not in my genes.

I'm sure I had my heart problem because of the extremely unhealthy life I had been leading. I started smoking cigarettes and a pipe at age 20, and even after I developed angina in 1965, I couldn't stop smoking. But in 1974 I developed a smoking-related cancer on the roof of my mouth. That was a terrible shock; only because of it did I manage to quit.

Furthermore, I was in terrible physical shape—and had been for thirty years before the onset of angina. I did not exercise at all.

For many years my way of life was stressful, to say the least. I chaired a large department at a local university and was president of a national society. Because I often had to travel to meetings all over the country, I found that I was continuously running at top speed through airports, waiting impatiently for flights, trying to find taxis—all, sometimes, just to give a brief after-dinner presentation at a banquet. In addition, of course, I had to do research, teach, and publish papers and books. I am convinced that the severe chronic stress that characterized my life was a major factor leading to my heart problems.

Another unhealthy aspect of the life I was leading was that I often had to entertain visiting colleagues, usually at gourmet dinners or lunches. Apart from the rich food, we usually had cocktails beforehand and wine with the meal. Even when I was not traveling or entertaining, I had bacon and eggs every morning for breakfast and frequently a steak at dinner. This diet, in conjunction with my sedentary lifestyle, resulted in a gradual weight gain, until I was at least 20 pounds overweight.

In 1965, at age 54, I began to feel a constricting pressure and tightness in the region of my breastbone whenever I walked. The pain went away when I stopped walking.

My physician referred me to a cardiologist, who diagnosed angina. During a routine physical, he also detected signs that my thyroid gland might be producing too little thyroid hormone; a blood test confirmed that he was right. This was unfortunate, I was told, because low thyroid hormone levels make the blood cholesterol rise. I was unusual, moreover, in that this particular disorder (Hashimoto's thyroiditis) is ten times more common in women than in men. The disorder was treated with thyroid pills.

The only other treatment the cardiologist recommended was that I keep a vial of nitroglycerine in my pocket and put one under my tongue whenever I felt chest pain. This, he told me, would increase the blood supply to my heart muscles by relaxing my coronary arteries.

He gave me no advice about diet or exercises and although he knew I smoked, did not advise me to quit smoking. In 1965 doctors were still unaware of the risk factors for atherosclerosis.

In February of 1974 my cardiologist referred me to a cardiac rehabilitation program. Before doing so, he said that researchers had begun to realize that a high-fat diet was bad for the heart, and he referred me to a dietitian—who informed me that everything I had previously considered food was now nonfood. The cardiologist also offered me a new drug, recently available, to combat angina; but I refused to take anything new and untried.

I thought the cardiac rehabilitation program was terrific and soon became friendly with all the nurses. The program was not always easy. The cardiologist told me to take a nitroglycerine tablet before exercising to relax my coronary arteries. The nurses had me jog around the track for a full thirty minutes, and when I slowed down, they urged me on, ever faster. At times I felt that they were sadists, asking a 63-year-old man to do too much. For the first couple of months, I was so stiff after those daily exercises that I could hardly walk. But the nurses were right and I was wrong. It took two years before I could exercise in comfort, but eventually I made it.

The nurses also encouraged me to stick to my new diet. This I really enjoyed, because I could tell what it was doing for me. I shed 20 pounds (9 kg) over a period of several months and have maintained my new weight for twenty-five years. The combination of a low-fat diet and exercise really works!

In March 1978, at age 67, the nature of my chest pain changed. The pain lasted longer and occurred almost immediately after I began walking. It also responded less and less well to the nitroglycerine.

The cardiologist said that what I now had was called unstable angina. He performed a coronary angiogram, which showed a complete blockage of my right coronary artery and a 70 percent narrowing of the circumflex and anterior descending branches of my left coronary artery. He referred me to a cardiac surgeon, who recommended a quintuple coronary bypass. The surgeon would need portions of five veins to bypass the blockage in my coronary arteries.

I was terrified of open-heart surgery; in those days it was still regarded as an unusual, high-risk procedure. When I told the cardiac rehabilitation nurses about my concerns, they got me to talk to others in the group who had had the procedure. These conversations helped to allay my fears.

But in many ways my fears were justified. After the operation I developed two serious complications. The first was a massive bleed in the area around my lungs; the surgeon had to open me up again to stop it. The second was ventricular fibrillation, during which the ventricular contractions became very rapid and uncoordinated: the heart doesn't contract, it quivers, and it can't pump blood to where it is needed. The intensive care nurses immediately used a defibrillator and saved my life. (Ventricular fibrillation is one of the main causes of sudden death.) Although I was also given quinidine to prevent fibrillation from occurring again, I had a severe adverse reaction, including high fever and a whole-body rash. All of these treatments had to be discontinued.

I vividly remember two other things about the surgery. The first was a severe pain in my breastbone, which the surgeons had to split in order to do the surgery at all; the second was the tube inserted down my throat, through my voice box, so that I could breathe but not speak. Although it was uncomfortable, I was terrified when they removed it, not knowing whether I would still be able to breathe or not.

After about a week I was moved from the windowless intensive care unit into a room with a beautiful view of trees and grass. Only then did I realize that I would be all right.

I attribute my recovery, from the surgery itself but also from the two complications and the drug reaction, to the excellent physical condition I was in beforehand. This in turn was the result of those exercises I had initially been so reluctant to do. They had come to seem a pleasure, and over the preceding four years had certainly made me more physically robust.

Upon discharge from the hospital, I began walking every day, and after six weeks I rejoined the cardiac rehabilitation program.

In 1986 my cardiologist retired, and I acquired a new, more aggressive individual. She refused to tolerate my attitude toward new medications—in fact, she read me the riot act. She insisted that I take medications to lower my cholesterol. The first was a drug that would, she said, absorb the cholesterol from the bile secreted into the intestines—the drug itself would never be in my bloodstream at all.

I found I could not tolerate this medication. It was as if I were drinking a mixture of water and sea sand; afterward I had to cough in order to bring the sand up from my throat. After trying various other cholesterol-lowering drugs, none of which I tolerated, the cardiologist eventually settled on one called a statin, which I have since taken intermittently. In addition, she increased the dosage of thyroid hormone I was on and prescribed a calcium channel blocker, which, she said, would lower my blood pressure and dilate my coronary arteries.

All was well until one Sunday morning in 1989, when I suddenly felt an agonizing pain in my chest. My wife rushed me to the urgent care unit, where the cardiologist on duty (not my usual cardiologist) did an electrocardiogram and blood tests for enzyme levels.

Both were normal.

Mystified, the cardiologist, looking through my very thick chart, noticed that in 1966 a barium study of my esophagus had shown that I had a hiatal hernia. Not unnaturally, he concluded that my stomach and esophagus were acting up again and giving me indigestion. Assuring me that nothing was wrong with my heart, he asked me to sit in the waiting room and see if the pain would diminish spontaneously.

Actually, the pain got worse. I felt extremely faint. Alarmed, the cardiologist examined me again; the only physical sign he found was that my temperature was rising. Baffled, he admitted me to a hospital, where he asked the radiologist there to take an ultrasound of my abdomen. He was thinking about gallstones, kidney stones, and other causes of sudden, excruciating pain.

What the radiologist found came as a complete surprise to the cardiologist and a shock to me.

The biggest artery in the abdomen is the aorta, which descends from the diaphragm to just above the pelvis, where it splits in order to supply each leg. The diameter of the aorta in my abdomen was 6 centimeters, twice as large as normal.

I had had, the cardiologist explained, an aneurysm, and the reason for my pain was probably that the aneurysm was leaking blood. Cholesterol, he went on, is deposited in the walls of all the arteries, not just those that supply the heart. This is what is meant by hardening of the arteries or, to use the technical term, atherosclerosis. Sometimes, when the wall of the diseased artery weakens and bulges, as in my case, the result is an aneurysm.

Since my aneurysm was already leaking, there was considerable risk that it could burst at any moment, with catastrophic consequences. My fear increased when the attendants came to wheel me into the operating room. There the surgeon and his team replaced the area of the bulge, down to the ends of the two main arteries leading to my legs, with an inverted Y-shaped tube made of synthetic materials.

My recovery after this operation was slower and more painful than after my previous heart operation. After eight long weeks, I felt that I had truly recovered. My wife and I decided that we had earned a vacation in a restful place, especially since it was our fiftieth wedding anniversary. We selected Canada and chose a lovely spot in the mountains, about 7,500 feet (2,273 m) above sea level.

The first night, after celebrating with a gourmet Italian dinner and a bottle of excellent red wine, my wife suddenly said that she felt very weak and that her heart was beating irregularly.

I rushed her to the nearest hospital and she was immediately admitted. The doctor there prescribed digitalis, which he said would control the irregularity and increase the pumping strength of her heart muscles. In the meantime, she was attached to an electrocardiogram, so that the nurses could monitor her heart rhythm continuously.

After several hours, exhausted after a busy and frightening evening, I retired to my hotel room. Unbeknownst to me, during the night my wife's electrocardiogram deteriorated and she was rushed to a much larger hospital.

When I went to visit the next morning, I walked innocently into her room. Her bed was empty, made up with clean sheets, and the closet, where her clothes had been, was empty. I panicked. I felt sure she was dead. But after what seemed an eternity, I found a nurse who could explain what had happened.

I rushed to the new hospital where, I discovered, the cardiologist had already done an angiogram and made a diagnosis. My wife, he said, had an overgrowth of heart muscle in the wall dividing the two ventricles of the heart, just below the aortic valve. When the heart contracted, the resulting bulge partially blocked the blood flow through the aortic valve. The muscle thickening, in addition, made her entire heart much stiffer; it relaxed less easily, which allowed even less blood into the heart.

He also said that the contraction of the thickened muscles of her heart was exaggerated anyway; but she had worsened overnight because of the digitalis received at the small hospital, which had increased the strength of an already overly strong heart, blocking even more seriously the blood flow through the aortic valve.

When we returned home, my wife's cardiologist confirmed the diagnosis, telling us that the official name of the disorder was idiopathic hypertrophic subaortic stenosis, which is abbreviated IHSS. ("Idiopathic" means the cause is unknown.)

I now worry continuously about my wife. Yet it is helpful to have two people in the same family working to control their heart disease, and my wife now also belongs to the cardiac rehabilitation program.

In 1997 I discovered that, during the rest period following exercise, my pulse rate dropped to thirty to forty beats per minute. My cardiologist gave me a monitor to wear for twenty-four hours, which confirmed that my pulse was very slow—problematic, as an extremely slow pulse rate can lead to cardiac arrest. So she inserted a pacemaker.

In 1998 I had two episodes of acute angina. On the first occasion, the cardiologist introduced two stents into one of my coronary arteries. After the second episode of angina, she put a stent into another coronary artery.

So here I am in 1999, thirty-four years after first developing angina, with a body that is walking testimony to modern medical procedures and devices: five grafts to bypass my blocked coronary arteries, a plastic tube in place of part of my aorta, a pacemaker that beats my heart for me whenever necessary, and three stents to widen my narrowed coronary arteries. Without all this technology I would have died long ago.

And because of my low-fat diet and my continuous participation in a cardiac rehabilitation program, I am 20 pounds lighter than I was twenty-five years ago and almost as fit as a healthy 60-year old. This combination of amazing medical procedures and devices, together with a cardiac rehabilitation program, has prevented my angina from progressing to an actual heart attack—and, in fact, my heart muscle itself is undamaged to this day.

What I Have Learned

After all that has happened, here is what I have learned:

- That my physicians prevented angina from progressing to a heart attack—by noticing that my thyroid gland was not producing enough hormone, later by means of timely bypass surgery, still later by insisting that I take cholesterol-lowering drugs, and finally by stenting my coronary arteries.
- That atherosclerosis affects all the arteries of the body (not just those serving the heart), including especially the

abdominal aorta, where I developed an aneurysm. Here again, timely surgery, performed just as the aorta was about to rupture, prevented potential disaster.

- That digitalis makes the functional effects of idiopathic hypertrophic subaortic stenosis, which my wife developed, much worse. It is a real comfort that both of us are in the same cardiac rehabilitation program, learning from and helping each other.

CHAPTER 8

Success without Angioplasty or Surgery

Jacob Gershon

After my heart attack many years ago, I soon found that no one was telling me what lifestyle changes I might have to make to keep from having another. These days, most cardiologists and other health professionals readily offer such advice, but that was not the case for me—and if you are in a similar situation, perhaps my experience can serve as a guide.

My heart problems began in January 1984, at age 51. I awoke one night with crushing pain behind my breast bone, which radiated up into my neck and jaws and later spread to both elbows and fingers. I saw my physician the next day. My EKG was normal. The doctor said that the fingers in which I had felt pain were usually involved in patients who had regurgitated acid from the stomach into the esophagus, but that patients with coronary artery disease felt pain in different fingers.

I had a particularly severe episode in early October of 1984. I woke my wife to tell her I thought I was having a heart attack. She called a friend, who happened to be a cardiologist, and asked what she should do. The cardiologist told my wife I was just having a panic attack. Yet for two weeks afterward I felt weak and listless.

On November 10 my wife and I took a long overseas flight, and shortly afterward I developed a high fever and rash over my entire body. I consulted a physician, of course, who diagnosed hypersensitivity vasculitis, an allergic inflammation of the blood vessels caused by the dramamine I had taken to prevent travel sickness. It took me about a week to recover.

I returned to the United States on November 24, arriving in Washington, D.C. The next day, I was walking down the street there when, abruptly, I had all the signs and symptoms of a heart attack. I panicked, for many reasons, but one was that I realized that I did not know a single doctor in the entire city. What to do? Suddenly I remembered a lecture I had heard years earlier, about how to get a doctor in a strange city; the advice had been to call the nearest hospital, request to be connected to the most senior secretary or the hospital administrator, and ask that person for the name of the hospital's best doctor. The lecturer, whose name I cannot now recall, said that such advice will almost always be competent. So I dragged myself to the nearest store, found the phone, called the nearest hospital, asked for the cardiology department, and got the name of the best cardiologist. I had myself transferred to his secretary, and asked her to tell him to meet me in the emergency room. I managed to hail a passing cab and delivered myself there. I later discovered that my anonymous lecturer had been right: my cardiologist turned out to be one of the best in the United States.

When I arrived at the hospital, the cardiologist confirmed that I was having a heart attack. Shortly after I was admitted, I felt dizzy and faint, though I was lying flat on my back. An intern rushed in, having heard an alarm buzz on my monitor, tilted the bed so that I was virtually upside down, and gave me some sort of shot. The next morning, during rounds, the cardiologist said that my faint feeling had been due to ventricular tachycardia, a rapid contraction of the ventricles independent of the atria. Left untreated in a heart attack patient, the tachycardia can lead to fibrillation and death, but the intern had given me an injection of lidocaine in order to reverse it. If I had delayed getting to the hospital by even twenty or thirty minutes, I would unequivocally have been dead.

These were the days before the advent of the fax or e-mail, so the cardiologist called my hometown doctor and asked him to send copies of my EKGs via express mail. The next day the cardiologist looked at those copies during rounds, then turned to me and made a startling assertion: my doctor had made a mistake. The EKGs had been positive all along. The cardiologist also believed that my so-called panic attack in October had probably been my first heart attack, and that this was my second.

Later that day, a strange thing happened: I had painful bladder contractions, but when I tried to urinate, nothing happened. At rounds the next day, therefore, I announced that I could not urinate, that I really, really, wanted to, and that I needed to be catheterized. Since I had turned out to be so sensitive to various medicines, I asked the cardiologist if it was possible that this too could be an adverse effect of the medicines he had prescribed. The famous cardiologist responded that he had used the same medicines for many years and had never seen this particular side effect. He and his team left the room; I could faintly hear them discussing me in the corridor outside. A young physician, training in cardiology, materialized in the doorway, did not enter, but yelled at the top of her voice that my problem was entirely psychological, and concluded with, "Just pee."

I still could not urinate, though, and the next day I was writhing on the bed in agony. Just before rounds that day, I called a friend, an expert on bladder dysfunction, to get his opinion; he told me that my problems were caused by the medicines I was taking.

When the cardiologist and his team arrived, I told them what I had done, only to be met with stony silence. A few minutes later a nurse came in, unplugged my telephone, and said that the physicians had ordered her to do so; the long-distance calls were too exciting for me and very bad for my heart. But a sudden thought, not easy given the overwhelming urge to pee, struck me: the urge to *pee* is very bad for my heart. I asked to speak to one of my doctors. When he came in, I said that the severe pain I had was upsetting me and was detrimental to my heart.

A few minutes later a urologist came in and said, without examining me, that I had a large prostate that was blocking my urethra; therefore I could not urinate and I needed to be catheterized. With the prospect of relief in sight, I told him that my own doctor had looked at my prostate a couple of months ago and found it to be normal, and I suggested that the bladder dysfunction might be due to the medications I was taking. "Never heard of that," he said and walked off.

Left to contemplate my own immediate, painful, and explosive demise, I was rescued by a nurse who came in to catheterize me. She drained a large volume of urine from my bladder. Finally able to speak, and think, with something approaching normalcy, I asked the nurse if she had ever seen a problem like this. "Oh, yes!" she said. "Many older men have enlarged prostates, but they don't know it till they come to the hospital with a heart attack, and then they can't pee." Yes, well, I thought, they had probably also had bladder dysfunction because of the medicines they were taking.

Shortly before I escaped this hospital, a special nuclear medicine study of my heart showed that the entire back wall was not contracting. The muscles there were either dead or stunned.

Stunned myself, I talked to another cardiologist when I got back home, who said she wanted to wait a few weeks before she did further X-ray studies of the coronary arteries. In the meantime I was to rest and not work.

My coronary angiogram showed that the coronary artery supplying the back of my heart was completely blocked, and the other artery was narrowed. But because my problem had been undiagnosed for a year, some of the fine vessels stretching from above the blockage to just below it had enlarged; my body had performed its own coronary bypass, and I did not need major surgery.

Now that I knew what shape my heart was in, it was time to find out about my poor bladder. I had what is called a urodynamic study, during which the urologist discovered that I had been right all along. My prostate was normal, not enlarged at all, but my urine stream was slow and weak because the medications I was taking were indeed affecting my bladder function. The local urologist said that he had seen this problem often; because few cardiologists involved with heart attack patients knew about it, the medications they were prescribing caused the bladder dysfunction.

With regard to diet and exercise following the heart attack, the advice my cardiologist gave me was simple and to the point: it was not worth trying any diets, since most people did not stick to them, and I should exercise a bit more when and if I could. But I realized that my life depended on the flimsy vessels that had managed to bypass the blockage in my artery, and that the disease that had struck that artery could strike those flimsy vessels as well. I decided to make major lifestyle changes and began looking for ways to do so. I discovered that the best advice can be found in health letters and books from places you have heard of: Harvard, Tufts, Berkeley, Johns Hopkins, the Mayo Clinic, the Cleveland Clinic, the *New England Journal of Medicine, Consumer's Health,* and *Nutrition Action.*

Later I heard about a cardiac rehabilitation program, so I looked into that. The nurses running this program said that every member had to be examined by their cardiologist consultant; they said he was a great man, brilliant and astute. This doctor did me a great favor by recommending that I attend a lipid clinic.

The lipid expert discovered that I had four genetic problems, each of which contribute to the chances of getting a heart attack. First, the size of my LDL cholesterol particles was too small; they could slip through spaces between the cells lining the arteries, building up inside the walls and causing inflammation leading to atherosclerosis. I also had elevated Lp(a) levels, ApoE4 lipoproteinemia, and high levels of the amino acid called homocysteine.

The expert said that small LDL particles were present in half of the men who had had heart attacks, and that 30 percent of people with heart attacks had high homocysteine levels. The fact that I had all four of these genetic problems increased my chances of having a heart attack by 1,200 percent!

My great-grandfather and my grandfather both died of heart attacks, and my father had a heart attack at age 63, although he eventually died of cancer at age 74. My mother's side of the family had no history of heart disease. The lipid expert commented that, clearly, I had a strong history of heart disease on my father's side of the family, from which I probably inherited these genetic problems.

The expert treated my LDL and elevated Lp(a) levels with niacin; folic acid and vitamins B_6 and B_{12} were prescribed for the elevated homocysteine levels. My LDL particle size is now normal, as are my Lp(a) and homocysteine levels.

In testing my blood homocysteine levels, the lipid expert checked twice. First, he obtained a blood sample after I had fasted for twelve hours (the usual way), but he also took a sample four hours after I had had an amino acid called methionine with a glass of water. After that test, my homocysteine levels were sky high—which meant, the expert said, that I could never eat meat, especially red meat, because it contains large amounts of methionine, which would raise my homocysteine to dangerously high levels for many hours afterward.

The problem was, he continued, that eliminating red meat also eliminated the main dietary source of zinc, and lack of zinc can lead to brain damage with memory impairment. To remedy this, he asked me to take 25 milligrams of zinc a day and, since I was still having episodes of irregular heartbeat, 500 milligrams of magnesium. A convenient way to do this, it turned out, was a supplement that contained calcium as well as these two minerals—all of which, he said, would be good for the heart and mind as well as the bones.

He also advised me to add one or two tablespoons of ground flaxseed (linseed) to my breakfast, because it contains alpha linolenic acid, which the body converts to omega-3 fatty acids.

These in turn have been shown to reduce irregular heartbeat. (He did not recommend fish oil, another source of omega-3 fatty acids, because he was concerned about their mercury levels.)

Finally, if I was still having irregular heartbeat, I should immediately eat a banana, he said, because it is high in potassium and magnesium. Or take half a teaspoon of a salt substitute that contains potassium chloride, dissolved in a glass of water.

He told me that people with APOE4 lipoproteins—like me— should avoid foods containing cholesterol, and saturated and trans fats, the type found in partially or completely hydrogenated oils or margarine. All three cause LDL cholesterol levels to shoot up. He added that statements to the effect that one egg three times a week is safe may be true for some people, but they were not true for many others, including me.

He gave me handouts explaining the genetic basis of the abnormalities he had detected in me. The genes for small, dense LDL particles and for APOE4 lipoproteins are located, for example, on the short arm of chromosome 19, near the LDL receptors, while the gene for elevated LP(a) is on chromosome 6.

He suggested I take antioxidants to prevent the LDL particles lodged in the walls of the blood vessels from getting oxidized and thereby setting up an inflammation. The prescription was for vitamin E, 800 international units a day, as well as vitamin C, 1,000 milligrams a day. (A nurse at my rehabilitation program subsequently told me that an article in the *New England Journal of Medicine* claimed that vitamin E does not prevent heart attacks.)

In the course of our discussion, the lipid expert mentioned that there is now some evidence that infection can play a role in initiating atherosclerosis, or in precipitating the rupture of the fatty plaque underneath the inner lining of the coronary arteries. Inflamed gums, for example, could be a source of infection, so he urged me to pay special attention to dental hygiene. *Chlymidia pneumonia* has also been implicated, he continued, which is why he had ordered special blood tests for me, looking for antibodies to that bacterium, and also a test for c-reactive protein. (Both of my tests were negative.)

Finally, he said there was a substance called L-arginine, found principally in tofu and soybeans, that protects the inner lining of the arteries. The downside was that it would take a lot of tofu or soy each day to get the correct amount; the upside was that pills were available, and he gave me another handout. (During a more recent visit he mentioned a special candy bar called the Heartbar®, which is fortified with L-arginine, as well as other substances advantageous to heart health, and is pleasant to eat.)

As I drove home, my head was spinning with all this new information; I was glad to have that pile of handouts lying next to me in the front seat of the car. Once I got home, I was able to read and understand my situation more fully.

When I went to my first exercise class, I was introduced to my classmates. Nearly all were highly successful people. I had read several studies which suggested that successful people had far better outcomes after a heart attack than the average man on the street, largely because they found out for themselves what lifestyle changes were necessary in order to prevent another heart attack.

With the help of the nurses, all of whom were superb and who taught us how to manage many of our heart problems ourselves, we became a very close-knit support group. If someone did not come to one workout, one of us would call to find out why. If someone was hospitalized, several of us would visit.

Next, I looked at diets. Almost every other month, it seemed, a new diet appeared, promising me that I would lose 30 pounds in thirty days, ream out all the fat in my arteries, have a better sex life, and leap tall buildings at a single bound.

I first tried the Pritikin diet. Before my heart attack, I was on a high-protein, high-fat, low-complex-carbohydrate diet, but on the Pritikin diet I lost 60 pounds (27 kg), and have gained none of it back. Then, a developing diet groupie like so many other Americans, I tried the Ornish diet. On both diets, though, my

HDL levels were dangerously low, while my triglycerides were dangerously high. My lipid expert (I was becoming an "expert groupie" as well) found the problem: both diets limited my fat intake to 10 percent of my daily calories, so, unbelievably, I was eating too little fat. He prescribed a Mediterranean diet, and within eight weeks my "good cholesterol" was way up and my "bad fat" way down. It was, I thought, amazing.

At about that time, the news broke that a glass or two of red wine a day makes HDL levels go up and protects against heart attacks. On that basis, my general practitioner prescribed that much wine for me each night. To his surprise, my triglycerides shot up and my HDL levels plunged.

Later, my lipid expert told me that for people in whom the triglycerides go up and HDL levels go down on a high-carbo-hydrate diet, drinking wine or other alcohol has the same result. This included me, so he strongly advised me never to drink at all. He went on to say that drinking two or more glasses of wine each day makes the beta-blockers, the calcium channel blockers, and the ACE inhibitors ineffective. These are all medications commonly used to treat heart attack patients, so drinking that much alcohol could interfere with the treatment itself.

Two recent events have reinforced my new ideas about diet. The first was that my 12-year-old dog, Shayne, became ill. My regular veterinarian said that he needed an expensive surgical procedure. But I took Shayne to a famous school of veterinary medicine for a second opinion. The professor there requested laboratory tests and ultrasound examinations of Shayne's liver and kidneys, which did indeed show severe liver and kidney disease. According to this professor, Shayne did not require surgery. The problem was that the dog food I had been giving Shayne had too much protein for an old dog, and the prescription turned out to be low-protein dog food. My immediate reaction: If the high-protein diet could harm the liver and kidneys of an older dog, what would a high-protein diet do to an old geezer like me?

The other incident involved a six-day vacation that my wife and I took, which involved an eight-hour train trip each way and a bed-and-breakfast. The only vegetarian food we could get on the train was vegetables sautéed in butter, and the situation with breakfast at the inn was similar. We managed to get omelets made from Eggbeaters, but despite our request, the chef always added whole-milk cheese.

It happened that just before leaving on this trip, I had had my blood cholesterol checked, and it further happened that by accident the nurse had filled out two requisition forms. Equipped with this second and otherwise unnecessary requisition, I decided to check my cholesterol levels after the vacation. My LDL cholesterol had increased by 75 percent. If I had had any doubts before, I had none now. Saturated fats and cholesterol were clearly harmful to me.

I had now succeeded in mastering three sides of the four-sided pyramid that leads to better cardiac health—exercise, diet, and cholesterol-lowering drugs. My ever-vigilant wife pointed out that what remained was my own type A behavior, so I joined a type A modification group.

The results of the studies done by Meyer Friedman and his colleagues astonished me. I had been reading that improvements in exercise, diet, and cholesterol levels could lead to improvements in the recurrent heart attack rate in the range of 50 percent; Friedman's results, though, showed that addressing type A behavior was much more effective than any exercise or diet!

One of the things that the Friedman program stressed was to try always to be on time—but if you were late, not to become tense or try to hurry. You would save only a few seconds, and the tension and the haste could cause a heart attack. I was reminded of my high school English teacher, who many years ago told a room of 16-year-olds who had just begun to drive that it was important to be on time, but even if they were running late, to observe the speed limit and never ignore stop signs or red lights. "Remember," he had said, "It's better to be five minutes late than sixty years too soon!" He himself died at a ripe old age.

Although it has been sixteen years now since my heart attack, I feel well, my body mass index is 23, my blood tests are normal, and my treadmill EKG is 12.9 mets and Bruce stage 4, the best for me since 1975. So I have managed to keep the small vessels that bypassed the coronary artery blockage healthy by making lifestyle changes. You can do the same.

What I Have Learned

After all that has happened, here is what I have learned:

- That I was correct when I decided on a rigorous cardiac rehabilitation regime. My cardiologist discovered that I had complete blockage of one major coronary artery and narrowing of another, but that new vessels had grown to bypass the blockage. Thus, in the sixteen years since my heart attack, I have had no further angina and am now fitter and feel healthier than at any other time in my life. Although I have not had a repeat angiogram, the results of treadmill tests suggest that my atherosclerosis has not worsened and may even have improved. The result is that I have had no bypass surgery and no angioplasty—both of which would almost certainly have been necessary were it not for my regimen of cardiac therapy.
- That since I received no advice at all from my own physician about risk factors leading to my heart attack, the most important steps I took when recovering were joining a cardiac rehabilitation program and subscribing to health letters.
- That I had several inherited lipid abnormalities, as well as a high homocysteine level, which explained my familial history of heart attacks and which were factors leading to my own heart attack at a relatively early age.

- That several popular diets do not work for me. Before my heart attack, I was more or less on an Atkins diet—which led to weight gain and high LDL levels. After my heart attack I tried the Pritikin and Ornish diets, which allowed me to lose weight rapidly but were dangerous because my triglycerides shot up and my HDL levels fell through the floor. I have found that the Mediterranean diet works best for me; it gives me the best lipid profile, and I have managed to keep the weight off.
- That it is important to order low-fat food and avoid stress when flying.
- That it was a blessing that my wife became involved in my rehabilitation. It was she, for example, who urged me to join a type A behavior modification program, something neither of us has ever regretted.

CHAPTER 9

Miracles Can Happen with the Two Ds

Verne Peters

What my cardiologist and I were looking at recently was as close to a miracle as most of us are likely to get.

We were comparing two coronary angiograms. The first showed that the openings of two veins used by the heart surgeons to bypass my blocked coronary arteries had actually narrowed by 90 percent. The second, taken five years after the first, showed that those radically narrowed openings were normal.

A miracle? Only apparently. This dramatic change occurred because I believe in two Ds: the danger of cardiac Denial, which can kill you, and the beneficial effects of Discipline, with which you can actually overcome the damage to your heart.

My story is a long one, with a troubled start—but also, for me, a lovely ending.

My first heart attack occurred out of the blue on November 5, 1981, just before my sixtieth birthday. My father had lived to be 83 and my mother died at age 76 of cancer; there is no history of heart disease in any of my relatives. Although I smoked a pack of cigarettes a day for twenty-four years, I had given them up twenty years previously. My blood pressure and cholesterol were normal, and I was not overweight. My diet followed then-current American Medical Association guidelines: some 30 percent of my daily calories came from fat. I rarely ate red meat and did not eat mayonnaise or eggs at all. Since I lived in the midpeninsula and worked in San Francisco, I commuted by train daily—but I got plenty of exercise. I rode my bicycle to and from the train station, a total of four miles a day, and walked to and from the train station in San Francisco, a total of three (very un-level) miles a day. So why me? No one knows.

I awoke on the morning of the fifth not feeling well. On my way home (on my bicycle) I felt nauseous and had what I thought was indigestion: as soon as I got home, I canceled the dinner engagement I had with a friend that evening; then I began to feel more and more nauseous and called my doctor. He said I should get myself immediately to the nearest emergency room, which I did; an electrocardiogram showed I was having a heart attack. I was admitted to the coronary care unit and treated conservatively: I was given ten days of bed rest and discharged. No angiogram was performed.

After an additional month, I went back to work. There a friend urged me to join a cardiac rehabilitation program, which I did. From the first moment, I thought it was absolutely terrific. What I liked most was the many friends I made there and the wonderful support group it rapidly became—this included the other participants, of course, but the staff as well.

In my opinion, one of the most rewarding aspects of the program is that many of us visit other participants in the hospital or at home when they get sick. Some members of our program have died of cancer since; their heart problems having been looked after, they are living longer and are susceptible to other diseases. I have always thought it was important to visit the dying. Some find it difficult, but to me it is a necessity. Because of this involvement, one of my classmates at the cardiac rehabilitation program has jokingly, but admiringly, called me Saint Peter.

For the past seventeen years, I have attended the rehabilitation program for an hour a day, six days a week, and I feel strongly that this D, Discipline, is crucial. I feel equally strongly that anyone who has had a heart attack should be in a rehabilitation program for the rest of his or her life. While there are programs that allow participants to remain in rehabilitation for one year, or two years, or (tragically) only a few months, I feel that such programs do a real disservice to their participants. Most of us need the Discipline that lifetime programs require.

My other D, Denial, is equally important. Many patients having a heart attack deny (or are fatally unaware) that it is actually happening and do not call 911 or another emergency number. This is one reason so many people still die of heart attacks. Fortunately, I did not have cardiac denial; I realized that something was seriously wrong, and I did something about it.

Those who go to the hospital with a heart attack can develop a second kind of cardiac denial: they deny that their heart attack was a wake-up call and go back to their old lifestyle as if nothing had happened; they still do not exercise, still indulge in high-fat food, and remain unable to handle stress.

Another form of cardiac denial is to deny that exercising too vigorously can precipitate another heart attack, which can be fatal. When people who have had a heart attack exercise too vigorously, the fatty deposit beneath the inner lining of the coronary arteries can rupture into the artery itself. A clot can form around that deposit, which may in turn block the coronary artery and cause the heart attack.

This is precisely what happened to me in September 1990. Despite my own precepts, the importance of the two Ds, I had a temporary lapse of judgment and developed some Denial, with disastrous results. I was doing very strenuous work in my garden, which I knew I should not do, but I thought I could manage it. Suddenly I had severe chest pains. I hurriedly contacted my cardiologist, who ordered an angiogram—which showed that one of my coronary arteries had closed completely. I was referred for a coronary bypass procedure, which was performed immediately. The surgical procedure, and my subsequent stay in the intensive care unit, proved to be problem free.

But the long-term outcome of the surgery was not as successful as my cardiologist and I had hoped it would be. On four subsequent occasions, each about seven months apart, my bypass grafts closed up. Each time, I had to have angiography, followed by angioplasty. My wife became desperate. She hated the long hours in the hospital awaiting the results of each new procedure, and eventually she urged that we do something to prevent these constant blockages. She was right; and fortunately, help was not long in arriving.

My wife read of a new program developed by Dr. Dean Ornish, which she urged me to discuss with my cardiologist. He was basically noncommittal: "I can't encourage you to be on this diet; it's much too strict and has too little fat and too little protein." But we decided to try it anyway. Our decision was not based on any lack of faith in the cardiologist, who was, I had always felt, a remarkable physician—extremely knowledgeable, conscientious, and thorough, willing to see any patient personally any time of the day or night or any day of the week, if necessary. Rather, my wife and I were prepared by this time to do anything that might halt the progress of my coronary artery disease and stop what seemed an endless procession of angioplasties.

As luck would have it, a local nurse was looking for a topic for a master's thesis in wellness counseling. She realized that the Ornish program, although excellent, was expensive and time-consuming, so for her master's project she decided to see if she could develop a modified and inexpensive Ornish program. She presented her idea to my cardiac rehabilitation program, which decided to cosponsor it, and they asked for volunteers to initiate this new project. My wife and I eagerly came forward.

After the program ended, my wife and I decided to remain on the Ornish vegan diet, limiting our fat intake to 10 percent of total calories, and we have done so now for five years. To stick to this diet did require the second D, Discipline, but the results were worth it. After suffering four bypass blockages on my previous diet, I had *none* on the Ornish diet, and, as my coronary angiograms demonstrate, my once severely narrowed bypass grafts now look normal. So miracles can happen, especially if we take responsibility for them ourselves.

Discipline has been required to get the most out of my cardiac rehabilitation program in other ways as well. I have attended all of the health lectures and all of the fat-free and easy-cooking classes.

About a year ago, the program began a unit in type A behavior modification. The therapist conducted hour-and-a-half group sessions every two weeks and prescribed daily drills to be done at home. Here again, Discipline played a key role: in order to modify our behavior, we had to practice every day.

I also learned that there are two bombs that can go off if we allow their fuses to be lit: preexisting coronary artery disease and cardiac denial. I was reminded often of a type A friend, who many years previously had been admitted to the hospital with a massive heart attack. Shortly after admission, he converted his room into a kind of office, making business deals, one after another, on the phone from his bed. He was in Denial that he had serious heart disease—and shortly after his discharge he died suddenly, of a second heart attack.

What I Have Learned

After all that has happened, here is what I have learned:

- That the Ornish diet works for me. After a bypass procedure followed by four angioplasties, this seemed like a miracle. Once I had been on the diet for a long time, it miraculously reversed the severe narrowings at the openings of the veins used for the bypass surgery.
- That I need Discipline in order to stick to the diet. I myself also need to be in a cardiac rehabilitation program regularly over many years, and practice religiously all the drills we were given in our stress modification group.
- That Denial is dangerous. I was unwilling to admit that exercising too vigorously could cause another heart attack.

But it happened, and it was the cause of the bypass surgery I had to undergo.

- That my coronary arteries recovered because of what I call my two Ds—the virtues of Discipline and the dangers of Denial.

CHAPTER 10

Young People Do Not Get Heart Attacks (WRONG!)

Sonny Adams

Heart attacks are for old people . . . the chronologically challenged!! That is what I used to believe. So why did I get my first heart attack in 1966, when I was still a month away from my fortieth birthday? And why did my son get a massive, near-fatal heart attack at age 42? Why did my father die at age 60 of a heart attack, and why did my three brothers all die of heart problems? My mother too had heart disease. At age 51, she sought medical advice for a bruised leg and died suddenly of a massive heart attack in the doctor's office. Weren't we always led to believe that women's hormones protected them from heart disease until later in life?

Knowledge of heart disease has advanced by leaps and bounds in the last forty years. A while back, I attended a lecture given at a cardiac rehabilitation program. The speaker said that an article in the *Journal of the American Medical Association* reported advanced coronary artery disease in soldiers killed in action in Korea. The average age of those soldiers was 22! We have learned a lot since the early fifties and sixties about how to prevent heart disease, and I am eternally grateful to my doctors for their advice on medical technology and pharmacology that have extended my life span.

I may have been much like those American soldiers in Korea.

When I was a child, my mother used chicken fat instead of lard for cooking. We ate fried eggs and meat and some vegetables, and I loved liver and onions. Our diet was typical of the times. We really had never heard about cholesterol or saturated fat. We ran and played basketball, baseball, and football after school, but the fats were beginning to clog our arteries. Many of those soldiers in Korea probably ate diets similar to mine, but one thing in my favor was that I did not smoke, as so many of those young soldiers did.

The speaker continued that this first, early report actually underestimated the age at which coronary artery disease began. He showed us the data and slides of a later study published in the *Journal of the American Medical Association*, which described autopsies on men and women aged 15 to 34 who had died in automobile accidents. The coroner found coronary artery disease in boys and girls as young as 15. A key finding was that the younger children had fatty streaks in their arteries, whereas young adults had hard plaques. Tests showed that fatty streaks often become life-threatening plaques later on. Clearly, the speaker went on to say, we need to teach even young children the benefits of heart-healthy eating and exercise.

Back in 1966, on that day a month before my fortieth birthday, I was playing tennis, when suddenly I felt incredibly weak. I lay down on the court. I was pale and sweaty, but I had no pain whatsoever. After a while I recovered enough to drive home. I walked upstairs and lay down on the bed, still very weak. Lying quietly, I remembered a young manager at work. One Saturday morning he had complained of chest pain to his wife, who apparently suggested that he see a doctor on Monday. That night he had died of a heart attack. I decided to call my doctor immediately, even though it was the weekend.

In those days doctors still made house calls, and mine appeared within a few minutes to examine me. He gave me the option of calling an ambulance or having him drive me to the hospital, and together we carefully descended the stairs to his car. After an electrocardiogram in the emergency room, the doctor told me that I was a textbook case of heart attack. I learned an important lesson: that heart attacks can be painless, because of something doctors call silent myocardial infarcts.

Rest was the prescribed remedy for a heart attack, and I remained in the hospital for three weeks. The doctor warned me that I had a 50 percent probability of recurrence of a heart attack within five years. (In 1966 a second heart attack was almost invariably fatal.) At that time, of course, there was no such thing as cardiac rehabilitation. All my doctor suggested was that I lose 10 pounds (I was then 170, having weighed 160 pounds at age 20) and take daily walks.

Today, thirty-four years after my "death sentence," I can look back and reflect on how fortunate I have been. Our understanding of the importance of diet, stress reduction, and social support has changed enormously since 1966. Internal medicine and surgery have taken gigantic leaps forward with regard to techniques, instruments, and medications. If I had to have a heart attack, I am lucky that I had it when all these changes were taking place.

Let me now describe how all those advances helped to keep me alive into the twenty-first century.

Six months after my heart attack, my wife and I thought it might be beneficial to my heart if I changed jobs. Since I was well qualified, an expert statistical engineer, I had no difficulty finding a new job doing classified ICBM (submarine missiles) work. My role, in fact, became pivotal: the success of the project was due in part to my knowledge of applied mathematical statistics. Every evening after work I would walk the neighborhood, away from telephones, television sets, and radios, a total of perhaps twenty to thirty miles a week. By the end of each walk, I was completely relaxed and rejuvenated. What those walks did for me mentally seemed, at the time, more important than any physical exercise I might also be getting. (When I later retired, I joined a local walking club, to extend the time I could spend on the nearby trails.)

I tried to reduce the amount of fat in my diet, especially of saturated fat. I drank only skimmed milk. I cut out desserts. My wife would occasionally eat beef and steak, but I went for chicken and fish. Also, much to my chagrin, my wife was and continued to be a heavy smoker. When we traveled by air, we always sat in the smoking section of the plane, and of course today we know that secondhand smoke can be dangerous to heart patients and others suffering from asthma. (The Environmental Protection Agency has classified environmental tobacco smoke a class A carcinogen, along with asbestos, benzene, and radon gas.)

My job at the time was becoming very stressful—not the technical part, which I found interesting and stimulating, but the interactions with some of the people. During the years 1966 to 1971, I felt very well and had no symptoms. But in 1971 I developed a bad cold, together with some chest pain, which was subsequently diagnosed as angina. When the cold disappeared, so did the angina; it did not recur until six months later while I was on vacation. When I returned home, my physician sent me to his professor for a coronary angiogram. The technique was very new, and a large contingent of medical professionals worked on me using this new technology. The results indicated that I would be a candidate for a coronary bypass, another brand-new procedure, but I did not like the risks involved. At the time, 15 percent of the bypass patients died! With no data to indicate whether the bypass would forestall future heart attacks or prolong my life, I turned down the surgery.

For the next five years, thanks to the latest drug treatments, I felt completely well. I experienced no angina. But then I did something that I now know heart patients should never do: I overexerted myself.

It was 1977. I was doing heavy manual labor, replacing the floor of my bathroom, when at 5:00 p.m. I suddenly felt chest pain. I lay on the couch to rest. Shortly afterward, my wife came home from work, and my son visited with a doggie bag of takeout Chinese food (which was delicious). After dinner, I went to bed with more chest pains. In the early hours, I awoke with excruciating chest pain and tightness. It felt as if someone was tightening a steel band across my chest, and I could not breathe.

Fortunately, we live only five minutes from the hospital, so my wife drove me to the emergency room. The physician took an electrocardiogram, which showed that I was in the throes of a heart attack. At that time, before calcium channel blockers and beta-blockers, cardiologists customarily waited 90 to 120 days after a heart attack before taking an angiogram. Returning to the same professor I had consulted in 1971, I learned that surgeons had gained valuable experience over the years, and the survival rate from a coronary bypass had significantly improved to better than 98 percent. I felt it would now be safe to have the operation. The triple bypass procedure, performed in April 1978, was a great success, but the cardiologist recommended that I stay away from work for an additional two months. Total recovery from the myocardial infarct and the bypass took six months.

When I finally returned to work, one of my coworkers, who had recently had a heart attack, told me about Dr. Meyer Friedman, who was recruiting people for a study of the effects of behavior modification on heart attack survivors. I could see from my own life how stress could affect the heart, so I enthusiastically volunteered.

Friedman's presentation impressed me enormously. In a previous study of healthy persons without heart disease, he had shown that behavior modification reduced their risk of heart attack by 200 percent. Dr. Friedman wanted to find 900 patients, who would be separated into two groups, 600 for a treatment group and 300 as controls. Both groups would get the same medical advice and treatment, but the study group would receive behavior modification therapy free of charge. Attendance was required at two one-and-a-half-hour sessions per month for five years, and videotaped interviews would take place at the beginning and end of the study. I fervently hoped I would be selected for the treatment group, and I waited anxiously before I learned that I had been accepted. I was assigned to a psychologist-led group to determine whether or not type A behavior was a major factor in recurrent heart attacks.

At each session our group was given a list of drills, which we were asked to practice every day for fourteen days between sessions. This I did, but it took several years before any behavioral changes showed up on a permanent basis, before I lived these changes automatically. Certain aspects that I have taken to heart (and that have helped my heart) include "Is it worth dying for?" (for example, reacting angrily when someone cuts me off in traffic), separating the trivial from the important, and ASAS (Acceptance of things as they are, Serenity, Affection, and Self-esteem). I learned that my life and my self-esteem had derived largely from my work, as I had always believed that this was the way to show love and affection to my wife and children. Furthermore, I learned to accept things as they are and not try to change the behavior of my family or other people. I learned to express my feelings openly and to listen to other people.

By the fourth year of the research project, the results were so dramatic in the treatment group—44 percent fewer heart attacks than in the control group—that the National Heart, Blood and Lung Association (which had funded the research) said that it would be unethical to withhold information any longer from the control group. The study was stopped six months early. I felt that I had benefited so much from the program that I decided to continue, and have done so to this day.

In 1992 my wife was diagnosed with pancreatic cancer. Fortunately, by then I had retired and could care for her in her last days. Her death came as a great shock, but I had learned to deal with all events more rationally. Time passed and eventually I fell in love again. My new wife embodied a lifestyle of more healthful living, which was helpful to me as well. And she had never smoked. With all the new health information available, it was easy to eat a low-fat diet of fish, skinless chicken breast, and a great variety of whole grains and fresh fruit and vegetables. It has served me well.

In April 1995 arrhythmia caught up with me, probably caused

by scar tissue from the heart attacks. For many years I had experienced an irregular pulse, which gradually deteriorated into tachycardia (fast rhythms). My cardiologist sent me to a specialist, who inserted a defibrillator—another example of technology available just as I needed it. My cardiologist and the specialist had trained together, and they communicate regularly about me and my medications. In my experience, it has been vitally important to be a *person* to my doctors and not a number! And I have benefited greatly from the teamwork I see in the medical profession.

At about this time, a physician friend of mine suggested that I might have high blood levels of homocysteine, now thought to be a major cause of heart attacks. On his advice I consulted a lipid expert, who discovered that I marginally fit into this category. The treatment was folic acid, in addition to which the doctor advised niacin, vitamins B_6, C, and E. These cutting-edge treatments have successfully reversed the lipid abnormalities that I had.

But the lipid expert was not yet through. His test revealed that my LDL, or bad cholesterol, particles were too small, which enabled them to slip between the small holes in the inner lining of the arteries and set up an inflammation in the walls of the arteries themselves. Moreover, I had high levels of something called Lp(a), a genetic abnormality of the LDL particles that raises the probability of heart attacks. No wonder both of my parents died young of heart attacks and that my son too has coronary artery disease!

Life continues with its ups and downs. The downs have been an angioplasty and stent, a pacemaker, and a radio-frequency ablation in the last few years. In general, life has been good to me. As I reflect on the thirty-four years since my first heart attack, I am amazed to discover that I have lived more than twenty years longer than my mother, thirteen years longer than my father, and twenty-eight years more than my original physician had predicted. I attribute this to my positive attitude toward exercise, diet, and stress reduction, but also to the enormous strides that medicine has made in the thirty-four years. For those, I will be forever grateful.

What I Have Learned

After all that has happened, here is what I have learned:

- That coronary artery disease starts in the teens and progresses slowly as we age.
- That my first heart attack was what is called a silent heart attack: I felt no pain at all, just extreme weakness and faintness. About 25 percent of heart attacks are silent and are discovered later because they cause heart failure or (less commonly) they are noticed on a routine EKG.
- That it was important for me to look into the possibility of inherited problems, because I had a history of family members dying from heart attacks at a young age. My lipid expert, in fact, found that I had inherited a tendency for small, dense LDL particles, elevated Lp(a), and heterozygous homocysteinemia.
- That it is vital to stay informed. I do so by attending lectures and reading health letters and other publications I have learned to trust. Only by doing this can I play an active role in my own health care.
- That the doctor who told me that I had a 50 percent chance of having a second, and fatal, heart attack within five years was wrong. The difference? My own positive attitude, a marked decrease in my type A behavior, and the enormous strides medicine has made in the last thirty-four years.

CHAPTER 11

Myth: You Are Lucky to Be a Woman

Joy Sing

The idea that women do not get heart attacks is a myth. Women get as many heart attacks as men; they just get them a little later in life.

A second myth is that Asians rarely have heart attacks. I immigrated from an Asian country, where a number of close relatives had heart attacks despite the fact that they were on healthy Asian diets. Several relatives on my mother's side have diabetes, and many have had heart attacks already, between the ages of 50 and 65—and some of my nieces and nephews have had heart attacks at even earlier ages. My own mother died of a heart attack at age 65.

A short time ago I went to a lecture on heart disease in Asians. It turns out that people of the Indian diaspora (from India, Pakistan, and Sri Lanka) have the highest incidence of coronary artery disease in the world. But more than 80 percent of those with heart disease have normal cholesterol! Their heart disease is due instead to genetic problems, involving small, dense LDL particles, low HDL2b levels, elevated LP(a) levels, high homocysteine levels, and—in many—insulin resistance, with high levels of insulin in the blood, leading to the development of diabetes.

Shortly after I arrived in the United States, I told my new physician about my strong family history of heart attacks, but

he gave me no advice about diet or exercise, or any other pre-
cautions I might expect to take to help prevent heart attack.
(Asian-American friends with family histories of heart attacks
have since told me that they had very similar experiences.)

I decided that I would have to provide my own preventive
therapy, and I reasoned that if I remained skinny, I would not
have a heart attack. I am about 5 feet (1.5 m) tall and have kept
my weight at about 105 pounds (48 kg).

About ten years ago, I had a blood test to determine my cholesterol level, which was at the upper limit of what that laboratory was then calling normal. After the famous Framingham
study was published, my particular laboratory decided to lower
its definition of the upper limit of normal. Given these new
standards, my blood cholesterol was now abnormal.

At menopause, which also occurred about ten years ago, my
physician put me on estrogen to prevent heart attack and osteoporosis. So at that point I felt extremely virtuous. Unlike my
mother and my other female relatives, I was very thin, I did not
have diabetes, and I was taking estrogens. I was safe: I would not
have a heart attack. I was wrong.

About eight years ago I visited my family in Asia. After I returned, I had a severe case of jet lag. I fell asleep while driving my
car. Fortunately, I did not run into anyone else, but the accident
was a severe one and I had a concussion.

For a year or so afterward, I was very lethargic. I thought this
was a side effect of the accident. In addition, my skin became
dry, my hair was falling out, and my eyebrows disappeared—all
of which were signs, I thought, that I was aging. When I asked
my doctor about these symptoms, he said that my thyroid gland
was producing too little hormone and that the cause was Hashimoto's thyroiditis, which occurs almost exclusively in middle-
aged women. One of its side effects is that levels of blood cholesterol rise (mine did, precipitously); at the same time, the level
of my HDL cholesterol plunged. This was serious, because even
small decreases in HDL cholesterol levels significantly increase
the risk of heart attack. My doctor prescribed thyroid hormone

tablets. But it took about six months for them to have full and stabilizing effects.

At about the same time, I noticed that when my hands and feet got cold, my fingers and toes became suddenly pale and then completely blue. When I warmed them, there was a strong reddish color. My doctor said I had Raynaud's disease, in which the small arteries supplying the fingers and toes spasm when exposed to cold. Women are affected five times more often than men. I was instructed to dress warmly and avoid exposure to the cold, and in addition to wearing gloves and mittens, to protect my body, head, and feet. One of the problems associated with Raynaud's disease can, on rare occasions, be spasm of the coronary arteries, leading to a heart attack.

When my family practitioner realized that my cholesterol was dangerously high and my HDL cholesterol dangerously low, she started treating me with niacin, which raises HDL cholesterol and lowers LDL cholesterol and triglycerides. But I could not stand the flushing and itching that niacin causes—and I developed a weird side effect, which my physician had never encountered: my nails became thick, irregular, and dark brown. They were hideous. So I begged her to give me something else; her choice was a statin drug. Although this lowered my LDL cholesterol and triglyceride levels somewhat, it had no effect on my HDL cholesterol levels, which were still dangerously low.

In January 1995 I developed chest pain while exercising. My family physician referred me to a cardiologist, who ordered a treadmill test, which he said suggested that my heart muscles might not be getting enough blood. The technical terminology was "a change in the S-T segment on the EKG." He stated that S-T segment changes give more accurate information about men than they do about women. For this reason, he decided to examine my heart during exercise, using ultrasound waves not electrical impulses. The result was negative. My cardiologist said that this result excluded any possibility of coronary artery disease, so he sent me home.

In June 1995 I left work early, at 3:00 p.m., to have my hair done. While driving to the appointment, I had increasingly severe chest pain. Remembering that the cardiologist had assured me that my earlier chest pain had not been caused by coronary artery disease, I decided to keep the appointment anyway. While I was at the hairdresser's, the pain became unbearable. I was alarmed, explained the problem to the hairdresser, and left before she had finished. Foolishly, I then drove home, instead of calling 911.

By the time I got home, I had no doubt that I was having a heart attack, so I finally did call 911. When the ambulance arrived, a neighbor rushed in to see what was the matter. I told her and asked her to notify my husband. In the meantime, the paramedics did an electrocardiogram, which confirmed that I was having a heart attack.

I was rushed to the emergency room, where the doctors gave me nitroglycerine to put under my tongue. The doctors also injected nitroglycerine into my veins—but the pain failed to disappear. I was clearly having a heart attack.

My own cardiologist, who by this time was present, ordered an emergency coronary angiogram. Three of my coronary arteries were very narrowed: one by 90 percent, one by 80 percent, and one by 70 percent. The cardiologist was shocked; only six months earlier he had given me complete bill of health. He turned to me and said I would need emergency coronary bypass surgery. When he showed me the angiogram, I agreed.

At this point I became very calm and relaxed. I am a deeply religious person, and I put my trust in the Lord to help me through this episode. (Later I learned that several studies have shown that religious persons fare far better during a heart attack than others.) I asked the nurses to try to contact my husband, who had not yet arrived despite my neighbor's efforts. I also asked them to contact my son; here I had more success, and he managed to be at my side almost immediately. In the fifteen minutes I had before the surgery was to begin, I told him all he would have to do if I died.

As I reflected on the fact that despite all the advanced testing, my coronary artery disease had escaped diagnosis when my symptoms first appeared in January 1995, I vowed that from this moment forward I would be assertive, taking responsibility for my own medical management.

I noticed that the surgeon who came to see me just before surgery that night looked very tired. I urged him to delay the surgery until the next morning. He agreed that he was exhausted and that he could do a better job after a good night's rest. But three of my coronary arteries were extremely narrowed and I still had chest pain. It was a life-threatening situation that required prompt action.

The surgeon had a solution. He would insert what is called a bubbler into my aorta, where the coronary arteries arose. This would force highly oxygenated blood, under high pressure, into the coronary arteries and prevent disaster.

As soon as the bubbler was inserted and functioning, my chest pain disappeared. I was proud that my assertiveness had worked. My decision might possibly have prevented unnecessary complications from occurring or even saved my life.

The bubbler made a continuous noise in my chest, which I could easily hear. The surgeon said that I would have to stay still and leave it on all night; turning it off for even a few seconds could have disastrous consequences.

At about 2:00 a.m. a nurse came in to examine my lungs. As she was listening to my chest with her stethescope, I noticed that I could no longer hear the bubbling and asked why. She said she had turned it off; she could not hear my breathing over all that noise. I told her emphatically to turn the machine on, that the surgeon had warned me that turning it off for even a few seconds could kill me. After the nurse turned the bubbler back on, she said that no one had informed her that she should not turn it off; in fact, she had planned to leave my room for a few minutes to get something she needed for me.

Taking charge of my own medical treatment had just paid off for a second time that night, and it has ever since. My recovery from this episode, and my state of health today, would be far worse had I not adopted this attitude.

My prayers were answered. The coronary bypass surgery was a success.

My biggest problem soon after the operation was that my left breast became very large and very painful. It was an awful sensation, and when the airway in my throat and voice box was finally removed so that I could speak, I asked the surgeons, during rounds, why this had happened. They told me that the breast is full of arteries, most of which arise from the internal mammary artery. During the bypass surgery, they had diverted this artery from my breast to my heart, so that it now supplied the heart.

Before my operation I had a wonderful voice, and singing in a choir had been a deeply satisfying part of my life. Apparently now, however, the airway in my throat and voice box had damaged my vocal cords.

When I was discharged from the hospital, the nurses and doctors gave me almost no instruction about cardiac rehabilitation. The little they did provide was nonspecific.

At home, my husband had bought me a treadmill so that I could exercise. I found a television program I liked and followed, but none of the exercises the handsome TV people did catered to the needs of heart patients. No one, for example, had told me that because heart attack patients are on beta-blockers, my pulse rate would not increase during exercise. The treadmill instruction book, for example, stated that I should exercise vigorously until I achieved my target heart rate, and a graph showed what that target rate should be. But, I later learned, the rates were not designed for people who had had heart attacks and were on beta-blockers. Determined to reach my target heart rate, I exercised on that machine until I was exhausted. Only later did I learn that exercising too much after a heart attack could have killed me. Excessive exercise can rupture the fatty plaque beneath the inner lining of the coronary artery, which can then protrude into the artery itself. A blood clot forming around that protrusion can block the artery, causing another heart attack, and sometimes death.

At about this time, a woman friend had a heart attack like mine. But this one was a puzzler: She was another skinny Asian, she did not smoke, she did not have diabetes, and her blood pressure was normal. A blood test done after she recovered showed that she had low cholesterol levels: a very low LDL (bad cholesterol), a very high HDL (good cholesterol), and very low triglycerides (bad fats). For obvious reasons, her doctors were puzzled; they decided to order a new test, which checked for levels of an amino acid called homocysteine. As it turned out, she had one of the highest levels they had ever seen.

In fact, a disorder called heterozygous homocysteinemia had recently been shown to be the cause of about 30 percent of all heart attacks. The treatment was simple enough: folic acid tablets. But her case underscored a vital point. Only one bio-chemical abnormality was enough to cause a heart attack, and that one problem had nothing to do with cholesterol or triglyc-erides.

In addition to the beta-blockers, my family physician pre-scribed other medications as well. The statin drug had a peculiar side effect: all my muscles became very weak. I could not, for example, even raise my arm to comb my hair, a symptom the doctor called a myasthenia gravis–like effect. So she switched me to another cholesterol-lowering medication, which I have tolerated well. I was also given vitamin E, an antioxidant.

My family and I have always followed a low-fat diet, but after my heart attack my family physician referred me to a dietitian— who told me to limit my fat intake to less than 20 percent of total calories and to take no saturated fats whatsoever.

As a result of all these measures, my blood cholesterol today is very low.

A friend urged me to join a cardiac rehabilitation program. And I am glad I did. The first crucial thing that I learned was that, because I am on beta-blockers, my target pulse rate during exercise should be low. (Had I joined the program earlier, I would never have done those possibly lethal treadmill exercises at home.) In retrospect, I cannot say strongly enough that anyone who has had a heart attack should be in this kind of program, run by experienced coronary care nurses. Without such programs it is easy to make a fatal mistake. Apart from the experience itself, and especially those superb nurses, I found myself making friends during exercise as well. This was an unexpected, welcome benefit.

Nor was this all. I eventually discovered something that became absolutely crucial to my continued health.

I had volunteered for a research project, during which my blood cholesterol and HDL levels were monitored at frequent intervals. I was amazed at the results. It was known that exercise could raise good cholesterol (HDL) levels, but most investigators thought that this occurred over a long period. But my results showed that whenever I traveled away from the cardiac rehabilitation program, or had a cold and did not exercise, my blood HDL dropped significantly and quickly. As soon as I returned to exercise, the blood HDL levels rose, as quickly and as dramatically.

These results have enormous personal significance for me. I had extremely low HDL levels before I joined the rehabilitation program. Since even modest increases in HDL can significantly reduce the chance of another heart attack, exercising at the cardiac rehabilitation program was literally a lifesaving experience for me. But I was also demonstrating, on a frequent basis, that those levels can change just as rapidly, and that no long-term process is involved. Exercise can help you recover from a heart attack right now.

Another difference between the exercises we do at the cardiac rehabilitation program and exercises people do on their own is that the program emphasizes stretching, to prevent injury to the muscles and joints. We also have exercises to strengthen muscles in our arms, legs, and abdomens, in addition to the normal aerobic exercises. In fact, we spend about ten minutes stretching and warming up before the aerobic exercises, and a twenty-minute section at the end is devoted to muscle strengthening exercises. I think our exercise is extremely well rounded, which is completely unlike exercises most people do on their own.

I find it most convenient to go to the class at the end of the day, after work, even though I am likely to be exhausted. Having people to talk to makes the class more entertaining—and the instructor helps as well, directing our next moves, giving us encouragement. I do not have to figure out the next exercise on my own. When I try to exercise at home, there are always distractions: the phone rings, my husband needs something, my son has a problem. So I enjoy exercising at the cardiac rehabilitation program, where there are no distractions, and no one makes demands on my time.

Despite the friendly efforts of everyone around me, it took a few months for me to appreciate all the benefits of joining a program. I did eventually realize how profoundly beneficial it is, though, and once I did, I invited a number of my friends to join up. Many happily remain, but some became discouraged after about six weeks and left. I discovered that those who left the cardiac rehabilitation program in fact stopped exercising altogether. For these and other reasons, I believe very strongly that a cardiac rehabilitation program should be a lifetime commitment.

My program has educational functions as well. There are two bulletin boards, on which the most important articles from that month's health letters are posted. I read them all, every month, because I learn a tremendous amount about myself and my body. I suppose it is possible for people not in a program like this to subscribe to health letters, but I doubt that any single person gets the large variety that the program obtains. Also, when the monthly bill arrives, it always includes invaluable health notes, which I have found that I enjoy reading.

I have taken many of the cooking classes as well, and have learned how to make genuinely delicious, fat-free meals that are easy to prepare. And I have learned a great deal simply by talking to other people in the classes. To me, the educational benefits have become just as meaningful as the exercises themselves.

What I Have Learned

After all that has happened, here is what I have learned:

- That women with coronary artery disease do not always have typical symptoms, and that electrocardiograms are more accurate in diagnosing coronary artery disease in men than in women. Women may need, not for the first time, to assert themselves in order to get good care.
- That when the surgeon diverted the blood supply from my left breast to my heart, the breast became swollen and painful. The pain and swelling eventually cleared up, but I suggest that women take a special bra or other breast support to the hospital, just in case.
- That decreased thyroid function is a major risk factor for heart attacks in women, because it elevates the blood cholesterol. Lethargy, loss of hair, loss of eyebrows, and dry skin are not merely signs of old age. They could be a result of decreased thyroid function due to Hashimoto's thyroiditis, which occurs almost exclusively in middle-aged women. My own doctor says that all women over age 50 should have their thyroid function tested every five years.
- That I should not try to reach the target pulse rate listed on my exercise machine. I am on beta-blockers, which slow the pulse, and too much exercise can be dangerous.
- That Asian diaspora Indians are at greater risk for heart attacks and should have their blood chemistry checked for small, dense LDL particles, low HDL2b levels, elevated LP(a) levels, and high homocysteine levels.
- That it takes determination, persistence, and time to make changes in one's lifestyle conducive to health. The effort is worthwhile.

CHAPTER 12

Risk Factors from a Patient's Perspective

Jerry Fox*

My story is vitally important for two reasons.

The first is that I was massively at risk for a heart attack. I had seven of the risk factors: I have diabetes, I had a strong family history of heart attack, my blood pressure was high, I led a very sedentary life, I was overweight, I smoked heavily, and I am a type A person.

Second, I developed a blockage of the large artery in the neck that supplies the brain, leading, in my case, to a mini stroke. (It is crucial to realize that heart attacks are due to rupture of cholesterol deposits beneath the inner lining of the arteries, and that the factors leading to those deposits can lead to similar deposits in arteries all over the body, causing loss of blood supply to other vital organs.)

My father, a diabetic, had a heart attack and several strokes and finally died of a stroke at age 64. My own physician explained to me that I had type 2 diabetes.

Someone offered me a cigarette at a party when I was 24—and I was instantly hooked. Within a few months, I was a three-pack-a-day smoker. But realizing that smoking was bad for me, I managed to quit, after a tremendous struggle, at age 50. I did not smoke again until I was 59—when someone, once more at

* Jerry Fox died shortly after writing this chapter.

a party, offered me a cigarette. And once again I was hooked. Smoking, we have since discovered, is unequivocally addictive. I smoked heavily, again three packs a day, for the next six years. When I think about the dreadful effects of that smoking addiction on my body, I am terribly angry.

After my first heart attack, my cardiologist told me never to smoke again, that smoking was the cause of 450,000 premature deaths a year from various causes.

About three years ago I became very breathless and developed a chronic cough. I was referred to a specialist in chest diseases, who told me that I had chronic obstructive pulmonary disease. Whereas my heart attack had resulted from several risk factors, one of which was smoking, this disease was caused by smoking alone. We have all heard about the link between smoking and lung cancer, but only rarely does anyone speak about the link between smoking and other equally serious diseases.

The chest specialist told me other things I will never forget: that 90 percent of those who smoke regularly become addicted, whereas only 50 percent of heroin users do; and only 10 percent of those who drink alcohol become alcoholics. Why? Milligram for milligram, nicotine is ten times better at making people high than heroin, cocaine, or amphetamines—and the nicotine in tobacco smoke increases the number of nicotine receptor sites in the brain by 300 percent.

When my diabetes first became evident, I was told to limit my sugar and starch. So I changed to a diet consisting, for example, of two fried eggs and coffee at breakfast, and meat and nonstarchy vegetables at lunch and dinner. When I had potatoes at all, it was in the form of a kind of pie called a potato kugel, made with eggs and a lot of chicken fat. I drank whole milk and ate lots of cheese.

So I was eating essentially a high-protein, high-saturated-fat, high-cholesterol, sugar-free diet with very little starch. And on this diet I became obese. This was unfortunate for a number of reasons: the former surgeon general, Dr. C. Everett Koop, has told us that three hundred thousand Americans die as a result of obesity each year.

After the heart attack, my doctor told me that diabetics need to keep their LDL cholesterol levels very low. Since eating saturated fats raises those levels, it was vital to eliminate them from my diet. My doctor prescribed the Reaven diet.

To make matters worse, I was getting no exercise—save only, prior to my heart attack, one game of golf a weekend. After the heart attack, my cardiologist told me that exercise helps to reduce insulin resistance, which gives rise to type 2 diabetes (the kind I had). The cardiologist also told me that exercising would be helpful in losing weight, which was important because excessive weight raises both the blood pressure and the LDL cholesterol levels.

When home computers became available, I spent all my time on-line, obtaining facts. When I became ill, I pretended I was a physician and used *Medline* (http://www.ncbi.nlm.nih.gov/ PubMed/medline.html) and other information systems to learn the details of my sickness.

To return to my health problems, about forty years ago I developed indigestion and heartburn. A barium Xray showed that I had a hiatal hernia and stomach ulcers.

I was treated with antacids, which reduced the symptoms for a time. Yet they always returned, and on two occasions the ulcers bled vigorously. Later I was told that the cause of those ulcers had been determined to be a germ, *Helicobacter pylori,* and the doctor treated them successfully with antibiotics.

During a routine physical in 1980, I was found to have high blood pressure and was given medications to treat it. Afterward, I was told that people with diabetes benefit from having a below-normal blood pressure, so I was given what is called an ACE inhibitor, to reduce my blood pressure and to protect my kidneys from damage due to diabetes.

On Memorial Day 1981, I had my first heart attack. My wife and I had been invited to a holiday picnic, but I did not feel up to it. The next day, I was completely exhausted; I had planned to work in my office but did not have the energy to get there. On the third day, I was at work in my office, popping antacids for what I thought was a recurrence of indigestion and heartburn.

I was wrong. It was a heart attack.

Since I did not feel well, I left the office early and called my doctor as soon as I got home. He told me to come to his clinic at once; I did, and an electrocardiogram showed I was having a heart attack. The doctor told me to call my wife and have her drive me to the hospital at once.

I was admitted to the coronary care unit, where enzyme studies confirmed the heart attack. After my wife went home, my daughter came and stayed the rest of the night with me. It was comforting to have her there, even though a handsome young medical student chatted on my bed with her until two in the morning, when I fell asleep.

It is difficult for me to understand how ignorant I was at the time about heart attacks. I did not know if my situation was life threatening or had the seriousness of a runny nose. The doctors gave me almost no information about what was happening. To someone who always wanted to know everything about everything, this lack of input was terrifying.

I found the coronary care unit a strange, eerily unfamiliar place. Bright lights were everywhere, twenty-four hours a day, making it difficult to sleep. The nurses questioned me hourly regarding the severity of my chest pain, and groups of medical students came at frequent intervals to put their stethoscopes on my chest.

After six days, the doctors posed one final test to see if I could be discharged. They had me climb up and down a flight of stairs and asked if I felt any pain. I did not, so I was able to go home where the lights were occasionally turned out and where, finally, I could get some rest.

It took me fully six weeks to recover my strength. Everything I did tired me. Still, I forced myself to walk a little longer, a little faster, each day—until, my proudest moment, I made it to a friend's house three blocks away.

Eight weeks after my heart attack I joined a cardiac rehabilitation program. One of the requirements at that time was
that all participants pass a treadmill test administered by the
nurses, and a physical examination by the program's cardiologist. I failed the treadmill test, and the cardiologist thought I
probably needed bypass surgery. My cardiologist agreed and arranged for my first angiogram, which was done by a cardiologist
specializing in the procedure, with my own cardiologist looking
on. When it was over, the two cardiologists looked extremely
worried and decided that they would *both* accompany me back
to the ward.

There, my cardiologist explained in great detail the risks and
advantages of bypass surgery. Listening to him and wanting to
get back to as normal a life as possible, I agreed to the procedure.
But I was definitely afraid that I would not survive it.

The heart surgeon, speaking with me before the operation,
warned that when I woke from the anesthesia, I would discover an unbelievable (to me) number of tubes in my various
veins and orifices. I would awake to a windpipe attached to a
respirator, which would pass through my mouth, throat, and
voice box. While it was there, I would not be able to speak,
and it would remain until I could breathe deeply and cough
to clear lung secretions. Another tube, a catheter, would pass
through my urethra into my bladder to remove urine and enable nurses to record my urine output. A third tube would pass
through my nose and throat to my stomach to remove stomach
juices. There would be two catheters in my veins, one in a neck
vein to measure blood pressure and the pressures in the chambers of my heart, and the second in an arm vein to administer
fluids, nutrition, and medicines. There would be two (or more)
tubes extending through my chest to drain blood and fluid from
around my heart or lungs, and, finally, my heart rhythm would
be monitored with a continuous electrocardiogram.

Immediately before surgery the ward nurse injected me with
a sedative. An attendant wheeled me to the operating room and
transferred me to the operating table, which was ice-cold metal.

My anxiety increased, and I was convinced these were my last moments on earth. A shiver ran down my spine, and my hands were clammy.

After the surgery, I was taken to a special intensive care unit for bypass patients. The surgeon told me that he had done five separate bypass grafts, and the tubes he had warned me about were all present and accounted for. The worst was the one in my windpipe, which caused the most horrifying sensation I have ever experienced. One particular nurse would come by and ask in a loud voice if I was having trouble with my respirator. I could not reply! At this point she would put a catheter in my windpipe and attach some kind of suction device. It felt as though she was pulling my intestines out by brute force. After three days, that tube was removed; and although, like everyone else, I resented the rest of my hospital stay, it was an enormous relief to have that instrument of medical torture out of my throat.

After I left the intensive care unit, I was taken to a large room with eight other bypass patients. Obviously, it was noisy and there was no privacy; but being able to talk to others who had undergone the same procedure was indeed helpful.

Upon discharge I was determined to rejoin the cardiac rehabilitation program, but it would be eight weeks before I was physically able to do so.

For months after the surgery, my wife had to put surgical stockings on my legs to prevent swelling, because the surgeons had stripped veins from my legs to use as bypass grafts. My resentment grew. For six weeks I could not drive, and toward the end of that time my growing hostility and type A behavior was surely evident to the world.

Once I did manage to rejoin the program, everyone welcomed me back in a wonderfully warm way. The nurses in particular were exceptional—kind, considerate, compassionate. I have no doubt whatsoever that they played a crucial role in my healing.

The people in my class were great, too. After each class, most of us went out for coffee, and quickly many of us became close friends. We had a kind of rotating dinner party at each other's homes. We also began to have a dinner dance once a year, then an annual golf tournament with a barbecue, and during the winter holiday season each class had its own holiday event. The friends I made in this way are still, after eighteen years, the closest friends I have ever had.

Ten years after my original bypass, I began to have angina whenever I went for a walk. The interventional cardiologist performed an angioplasty, but warned me that my bypass grafts could shut off again in three to six months. (They actually remained open for about three years.)

After the three years, I developed angina once again and was referred for a second bypass operation. This second experience paralleled the first but was much more taxing because I was older, and the recovery time was much slower.

Two years later, I was driving to a friend's house when suddenly a large gray blotch concealed the vision in my left eye. When I arrived at my friend's house, the blotch had disappeared, though I immediately called my doctor, who ordered an ultrasonographic examination of the big arteries in my neck.

The ultrasound showed that the artery on the left side of my neck was almost completely blocked. My doctor explained that the coronary arteries are not the only ones affected by cholesterol deposits; atherosclerosis is a diffuse disease that affects all the arteries in the body. It is vital that heart attack patients understand this.

My cardiologist referred me to an old-time vascular surgeon. Instead of cheerily sticking his head in the door and asking how I was, as most young surgeons today seem to do, he took the time each day to give me a thorough physical examination. I was overwhelmed with his excellence: he was thorough, kind, and patient, in the way we all want physicians to be. I was touched and amazed.

A few months ago, a spot appeared on one of my lungs on a routine chest Xray. My chest specialist said it was too dangerous to do a needle biopsy of that spot, because of my severe chronic obstructive pulmonary disease. He suggested that we wait three months to see what would happen. By that time a large number of spots had appeared in my lungs, and in my bones as well. The chest specialist did a needle biopsy of one of my ribs (safe, he said, because the needle would not go into my lungs) and found that I had kidney cancer.

I sat down in front of my computer and checked on the Internet, discovering that if there had been only a spot or two on my lungs, removal of the affected kidney and lung spots might cure the disease. But my chronic obstructive pulmonary disease precluded a needle biopsy when it might have done some good, as well as the surgery that could have saved my life. My smoking habit had delivered the final fatal blow.

I wanted to call my cardiologist regarding changes in my prescriptions, but I spent hours on the phone trying to reach him. I eventually discovered a simple solution, which I would like to pass on: now I send him an e-mail or a fax. Either way, I retain a hard copy for my records, and the end result has been dramatic. My cardiologist always responds as rapidly as possible.

What I Have Learned

After all that has happened, here is what I have learned:

- That milligram for milligram, the nicotine in tobacco smoke is the most addictive drug in the world, and tobacco smoke can have effects that go beyond cancer of the lungs. It can lead to chronic obstructive pulmonary disease, which, I can tell you, is like being continuously tortured. And, of course, smoking is the leading risk factor for coronary artery disease.
- That the most suitable diet for me is the Reaven diet. Prior to my heart attack, my diet had been closer to the Atkins diet, but it had resulted in my gaining weight, one of the risk factors leading to my heart attack.
- That I have benefited enormously from exercising in a

cardiac rehabilitation program—and that the nurses there have played a crucial role in my healing process.

- That a cardiac rehabilitation program is not just about exercise. I know that I have gained just as much from the people, the social support, and the friends I have made in the program. My best friends, really my only friends, are those I found in my program. Now that I am dying, they visit me frequently. One of them, whom we all call Saint Peter, is here constantly, comforting me and helping me to feel content and peaceful in light of the inevitable.

PART III

The Health Professionals' Perspectives

CHAPTER 13

The Complexities of Proper Nutrition

Christopher Gardner

Nutrition—what you eat, and how what you eat becomes *you* —is extraordinarily complex, and no one knows all the answers. What is clear is that no single diet works for everyone. Just as there are many components of good health, there are many different diets and each is appropriate for different people.

People with heart disease tend to ask similar questions about diet. Are there specific diets that are helpful to people with heart disease, including those with diabetes? Which diets will help to lose weight? What about the new medical foods, such as the Heartbar®? Are diets useful for treating heterozygous homocysteinemia? Will eating certain phytochemicals (plant chemicals that are not vitamins or minerals) prevent another heart attack? Which antioxidant foods are advisable, and will they prevent another heart attack?

The answer to the first question is yes, there are. Healthful diets for people with heart disease include the extremely low-fat varieties (the Pritikin, Ornish, and McDougall diets); those higher in unsaturated fats (the Reaven and Mediterranean diets); and, perhaps for short periods of time but not long term, the high-protein varieties (the Sears and Atkins diets).

How do we know these diets will help?

Studies are ongoing and are generally of two kinds. The first involves very large populations. Ancel Keys, for example, of the

University of Minnesota, first noted in 1970 that the two countries with the least heart disease were Japan and Crete. The fat content of food was very low in Japan, whereas Cretans ate considerably more fat than other populations, although most of that fat was unsaturated. What was similar in Japan and Crete was the low intake of saturated fat. Notably, the rates of heart disease are on the rise in both Japan and Crete, as the two cultures continue to adopt aspects of a Western lifestyle, including higher levels of saturated fats. Heart disease levels are highest in Finland and the United States, where most of the fat consumed is saturated, the variety found in meat and dairy products.

Such population studies are vitally important. Different eating habits among populations in various countries, measured over decades (and in some cases over hundreds or even thousands of years), can indicate the influence of diet on the prevalence of heart disease. Such studies, while helpful for indicating trends and generating hypotheses, are subject to a major limitation, however. They cannot distinguish between diets that are healthy and the possibility that people who eat certain diets are healthier to begin with, or follow other lifestyle practices responsible for their good health. Thus, other research is necessary to understand the links between diet and health.

This second type of study involves short-term clinical trials, in which researchers control exactly what people eat, then do blood tests to determine the effect of foods on *markers,* or risk factors of heart disease, such as total, HDL, and LDL cholesterol levels, as well as triglycerides. In this type of study, scientists obviously have more control over the conditions and are able to determine the effect of diet on health.

The problem in this type of study is that any one such trial gives only a glimpse of the answer. Typically, *one* isolated nutrient (say, vitamin E) is provided in *one* specific dose, to *one* specific and relatively small group of individuals (for example, one hundred men who have had a heart attack), for *one* duration of time (for instance, one year), to look at *one* or a limited number of health concerns (perhaps antioxidant status or recurrent heart disease). What cannot be addressed is the effect of a different nutrient, a different dose, given to a different group of people, for a different length of time, on a different health outcome. Therefore, any single study has many pitfalls, and many questions remain unanswered. Thus, the pieces of a complex puzzle must be put together one at a time.

Some Nutrition Basics

Getting Calories from Carbohydrate, Fat, and Protein

Most of the popular diets for people with heart disease, or for people who wish to prevent heart disease, attempt to control either the amount of fat or the amount of protein, which in turn affects the amount of carbohydrate that can be eaten. To see how these diets work, let us look at how the body handles these three main sources of calories: carbohydrates, fat, and protein. (Alcohol is a fourth, minor source of calories.)

The diets of most people in the world consist largely of carbohydrates. But there is so little space in your body to store carbohydrates—in your liver and in your muscles—that you can fill the available space with just one meal. The carbohydrates that you cannot store this way, or use immediately, are converted and stored in your body as fat.

When you eat fat, on the other hand, your body burns some of it right away but stores the rest. Unlike the situation with carbohydrates, your body has an almost infinite storage capacity for fat. Despite the well-known downside of too much body fat, there is a very practical side to your body's ability to store fat; it is a concentrated source of energy, it takes up less room and weighs less than storing carbohydrate, and it is simply efficient (when not overused).

Your body gives proteins, unlike carbohydrates and fat, no storage space at all. All the proteins you eat are used—to make hormones, enzymes, skin, nails, and muscles. We all need it, therefore, every day; but surprisingly, we need very little, only about 5 percent of our daily calories. Even bodybuilders need very little. If you wanted to increase your muscle mass by 20 pounds (9.1 kg) a year, about 10 grams of extra protein a day could do the trick (70 percent of lean tissue, or muscle mass, is water). This amount is trivial, considering that the average American consuming 100 grams of protein daily is already getting at least 50 grams per day more than is required.

Carbohydrates, fat, and protein are all composed mainly of carbon chains with hydrogen and oxygen. Protein also contains some nitrogen. As soon as the protein has met the functional needs of your body, the amino acids, which are the building blocks of all proteins, are broken down into their constituent parts, a carbon portion and a nitrogen portion. The carbon portion is converted into carbohydrate (for energy right away, or to replenish the body's carbohydrate stores) or turned into fat and either burned immediately or stored as fat. The nitrogen becomes ammonia, which is toxic to the body and is sent to the liver. There it is converted to urea, then excreted by the kidneys. So the more protein you eat, the more ammonia and urea your body will produce. This may be very important, as we shall see shortly.

The Role of Insulin

Nearly all diet books claim that their particular diet influences how much insulin the pancreas produces. To evaluate this claim, we need to see what stimulates the pancreas to produce insulin, and what insulin does in the body.

In general, insulin makes the muscles take up glucose after a meal and prevents the fat cells from releasing free fatty acids.[1]

In the morning, before breakfast, insulin levels are very low — which means that the muscles are taking up almost no glucose. Therefore, fat cells are releasing free fatty acids which, at this point in the morning, are the main source of energy for the heart and other muscles.

Eating carbohydrates or protein raises the blood glucose

level; eating fats does not. So after a breakfast of carbohydrates or proteins or both, glucose and insulin levels rise and the insulin starts putting glucose back into the muscles, where it is stored or burned for energy. At the same time, these rising insulin levels prevent the fat cells from releasing free fatty acids.

Apart from producing energy first thing in the morning, free fatty acids in the blood make the liver produce triglycerides. There is an inverse relationship between the blood level of triglycerides and HDL (good) cholesterol; when triglyceride levels are up, HDL cholesterol levels fall.

Sixty million to 75 million Americans who do not have diabetes do have what is called insulin resistance.[2] In these people, the pancreas secretes sufficient insulin, but the cells of the muscles are resistant to it, so the pancreas secretes more and more insulin in an effort to force glucose into the muscle cells. If this extra insulin manages to keep the blood glucose levels in the upper normal range (a fasting glucose level of 110–126 mg/dL), diabetes does not occur.

Such people also have "impaired glucose tolerance," in that their blood glucose level is between 140 and 200 mg/dL two hours after drinking water containing 75 grams of glucose. (The normal level after two hours would be less than 140 mg/dL of glucose.)

Insulin resistance is the result of three factors. About 50 percent of the cause is genetic (people who, genetically, are unusually prone to insulin resistance include American Indians, South Asian Indians, Japanese Americans, African Americans, Australian Aboriginals, and various Pacific Island populations), about 25 percent is obesity, and the final 25 percent is lack of exercise. We cannot, clearly, choose our parents. But we can control our diet and exercise.

Continuously high blood insulin levels can produce signs and symptoms that, together, represent a major cause of heart attacks. This group of symptoms has been variously called the metabolic syndrome, syndrome X, or the Reaven syndrome. Its symptoms include triglyceride levels of 200 mg/dL or more; HDL levels below 35 mg/dL; blood pressure greater than 140/90 mmHg; small, dense LDL particles; rising levels of triglyceride-rich lipoproteins in the blood after a meal, which remain high for many hours; high blood levels of plasminogen activator inhibitor-1 (which reduces the body's ability to break up blood clots); and high blood levels of uric acid (which may cause attacks of gout).

Reaven and colleagues point out that heart disease is twenty times more likely to occur in men with syndrome X than in the general population. In fact, a study in Quebec found that nearly 70 percent of heart disease victims had syndrome X.

If the pancreas secretes more and more insulin because the glucose has trouble getting into the muscle cells and cannot keep up, the fasting blood glucose level rises above 110 mg/dL, and the blood glucose level rises to more than 200 mg/dL two hours after drinking water containing 75 grams of glucose. This, by definition, is type 2 diabetes.

The Role of Dietary Fats

Many diets attempt to control the type and quantity of fats you eat. The two major categories of fat contained in the foods we eat are saturated and unsaturated fat. The unsaturated fat category can be further subdivided into monounsaturated and polyunsaturated fat. And even the polyunsaturated category can be further divided into fats derived from plant-based foods (sometimes called n-6 or omega-6 fatty acids) and those derived from fish and other marine-based foods (sometimes called n-3 or omega-3 fatty acids). Another category of fats that has received considerable attention in scientific studies and in the media is trans fat. Although technically a monounsaturated fat, it acts more like a saturated fat.

Large amounts of saturated fat occur mainly in food derived from animals: whole-fat cheese, milk, butter, and meat. Some plant products are also rich in saturated fat, including coconut and coconut oil and palm and palm kernel oil. The less saturated fat you eat, the better. Saturated fat raises LDL and total cholesterol levels, which can lead to atherosclerosis.

Monounsaturated fats are found in many foods, but predominantly in olive, canola, and peanut oils, and in most nuts. From the point of view of heart disease, monounsaturated fats provide at least two benefits: they lower LDL cholesterol in themselves and prevent HDL from being oxidized.

Polyunsaturated fats are also found in many foods, but predominantly in safflower, sunflower, and soybean oils, soy products, walnuts, whole-grain products such as whole-wheat bread, and fish. Of all the types of fat found in the diet, this is the only one considered "essential"—meaning that, your body cannot make it on its own, and adverse health consequences will result if you fail to get some in your daily diet. (Your body does make saturated and monounsaturated fat every day from carbohydrate and excess protein.) The amount of polyunsaturated fat that you need in your diet is only 2 percent of your daily calories, and deficiencies are extremely rare.

From the point of view of heart disease, polyunsaturated fats help to lower total and LDL cholesterol when they replace saturated fats in the diet. They also provide the building blocks for hormone-like substances that help regulate blood pressure and blood clotting. The types of polyunsaturated fats found in fish are particularly effective at lowering triglyceride levels; they may also prevent some kinds of irregular heartbeats.

Clear and undisputed heart benefits result from switching from saturated fats to unsaturated fats. In food language, this means replacing meat fat, chicken fat, and dairy fat with nuts, seeds, nut and seed butters, avocados, soy products, and vegetable oils. Any further benefits to be gained from choosing between mono- and polyunsaturated fat sources (olive oil vs. soybean oil, almonds vs. walnuts, avocados vs. sunflower seeds) are of smaller magnitude and may depend on individual characteristics, such as antioxidant status, blood pressure, blood coagulation status, and triglyceride levels.

Trans fats are more similar to the saturated fats they resemble than to the unsaturated fats from which they derive. They increase total and LDL cholesterol levels, and decrease HDL cholesterol levels. Trans fats are created by converting vegetable oil to solid or semisolid margarine, through a process known as hydrogenation. Soft or liquid margarines have very low levels of trans fats, but the more solid and butter-like the margarine, the higher the level of trans fats.

The media attention given to the "trans fat scare" has generated a great deal of frustration among those who at one point had switched from butter to margarine for health reasons, and felt that the new recommendation was to switch back to butter. That really was not the intended message. In order to make your own decision about the impact of margarine on your health, consider the following three possibilities:

1. Are you using margarine to replace butter? Since the total amount of saturated fat and trans fat in margarine is usually somewhat less than in butter, the net effect probably favors margarine when it comes to your blood cholesterol levels.
2. Are you using margarine to replace vegetable oils? If so, poor choice. The unsaturated fats in the vegetable oils from which trans fats are derived are healthier for you than the margarine.
3. Are you simply adding margarine to your diet, and not replacing any other sources of fat? Again, poor choice. You have just added calories and cholesterol-raising saturated and trans fat to your diet.

The bottom line is that trans fats are not a "healthy choice." But most people face decision 1 above; very few are thinking about decision 2 or 3. In that case, margarine is probably still a healthier choice, or at least no worse, than choosing butter. On the other hand, if you really prefer the taste of butter, then the health benefits of margarine over butter may not be sufficient to sacrifice your taste buds. As is often the case in nutrition issues, your best bet with either butter or margarine is to practice moderation.

Two final facts on the trans fats. First, margarine producers in the United States have taken the findings about trans fats to heart (pun intended) and have followed the lead of European producers by changing manufacturing procedures and lowering the trans fat content of margarines. Second, the major contributor of trans fat in the diets of many Americans is not margarine, but snack foods made with hydrogenated or partially hydrogenated fats. The snack foods therefore contain a double whammy: the trans fats *and* usually lots of sugar with low levels of nutrients compared to what else you might be snacking on.

It is, therefore, important to look at the food label for the total grams of fat, grams of saturated fat, and whether any fat has been partially or completely hydrogenated. The quantity of fat consumed is also critical. A meal, for example, in which fat makes up more than half of the total calories may be dangerous in people with preexisting coronary artery disease, even if they have no symptoms.

The dangers are several. First, a high-fat meal raises the levels of something in the blood called factor VII, which makes the blood clot. Factor VII may take six to nine hours after a high-fat meal to reach its maximum blood level, after which the level gradually falls. But this means that a clot in an atherosclerotic coronary artery may form hours after the high-fat meal, and the association may not be recognized. A 1999 study suggested that olive oil causes the least elevation of factor VII levels, which may be why olive oil is advisable for eating and cooking.[3]

A second danger of high-fat meals is that they may cause sludging of the red cells (see below).

Popular Diets

With all this in mind, let us look at the pros and cons of the most popular diets used today by people with heart disease (Table 2).

Table 2. A summary of diets for your health.

Diet	Advantage	Disadvantage
Very low fat	Avoids "sludging" or elevation of factor VII after a meal Weight loss Ornish version occasionally reverses coronary artery disease	Unsuitable for diabetics and people with syndrome X Elevates triglycerides and lowers HDL in some people, Can be hard to follow McDougall diet lacks vitamins B_{12} and D
AHA revision 2000	Looks at the big picture, not at individual nutrients Provides different guidelines for healthy people versus those with heart disease, high blood pressure, high cholesterol, syndrome X, or diabetes	People with heart disease, high blood pressure, high cholesterol, syndrome X, or diabetes may need medical and nutrition professionals to help plan and monitor their diet
Reaven	Highly effective in diabetics Prevents bloodstream lipids from rising after a meal	Provides only 500 mg of calcium a day
Mediterranean	Potential for fewer recurrences of heart attack (Lyon trial) Rich in antioxidants, phytochemicals, vitamins, fiber, and unsaturated fats Does not elevate triglycerides or lower HDL Usually thought to be delicious	Some potential for weight gain
High protein	Weight loss possible	Recommended for short term only (potential for liver damage) Atkins and Protein Power diets high in saturated fats and cholesterol Atkins and Protein Power diets high in methionine, which could raise blood homocysteine levels

Extremely Low Fat Diets

The extremely low fat diets (the Pritikin, Ornish, and McDougall diets) have two common features: they would have you derive only about 10 percent of your calories from fat, and all are plant based.

The term "plant based" merits discussion here.[4] It is being used more and more by nutritionists, but may not be familiar to others. A plant-based diet is similar to a vegetarian diet, but with an important distinction. A plant-based diet mainly contains vegetables, whole grains,[5] and legumes.[6] It is a high-fiber diet rich in phytochemicals and antioxidants, as well as other nutrients that may protect you against heart disease. In fact, a recurring theme is beginning to emerge: all healthy diets seem to be plant based. A vegetarian diet simply means that no meat is included. It is not necessarily a healthy way to go; a vegetarian could, in theory, eat jellybeans and cheese three times a day and be severely malnourished.

Pritikin and McDougall (but not Ornish) originally developed their diets because red blood cells tend to clump together as they pass through very small arteries, after even a single high-fat meal. This process, called sludging or rouleau formation, tends to block those arteries, a fact discovered by examining the conjunctival arteries before and after high-fat meals.[7] (It is presumed that this blockage occurs in the small arteries bypassing narrowed coronary arteries as well.) The blockage was found only in people with proven type A behavior who have had a very high fat meal. The sludging reaches its maximum about four hours after such a meal. Two participants in the original study, both of whom had had previous heart attacks but were currently symptom free, developed severe angina three hours after a very high fat meal. They were immediately treated by injection of heparin into a vein, with instant relief of symptoms and resolution of the red cell sludging.

There are significant differences among these diets. The Pritikin diet,[8] for example, allows lean red meat, skinless chicken breast, and fish, whereas the Ornish diet[9] is lactovegetarian and allows no meat, poultry, or fish. It does allow fat-free milk products, such as fat-free yogurt, as a source of vitamin B_{12}. The McDougall diet,[10] on the other hand, is vegan—based on whole grains, legumes, and vegetables—and allows little or no dried or fresh fruit (which is high in fructose) and no added sugar. Anyone on this diet will not get enough vitamin B_{12}, which can result in anemia, so if you decide to follow it, you will need to eat fortified cereals, drink soy milk fortified with vitamin B_{12}, or consider taking a vitamin supplement.

Dean Ornish has developed a program that has been successful in reversing heart disease in some people and successful with others in losing weight, apparently because high fiber and complex carbohydrates, in which the diet is rich, make people less hungry. But the total Ornish program involves significant exercise as well as stress reduction, which makes it hard to say whether it is the exercise, the stress reduction, the diet, or some combination of the three that leads to the reversal or lack of progression of the coronary artery disease. Despite my reservations, two of our contributors did report dramatic results. Once she was on the Ornish diet, Helen L'Amoreaux's angina disappeared, amazingly, after nineteen years (Chapter 5); and the two veins used by surgeons to bypass Verne Peters' blocked coronary arteries, which were 90 percent closed, were completely open after he too went on the Ornish diet (Chapter 9).

Still, the Ornish diet has limitations. It is so low in fat that it can be difficult to follow; it takes a lot of time to find and prepare the types of meals recommended. Few of us have that discipline; those who do are often ready to make other radical lifestyle changes as well, such as a significant increase in exercise level and attending stress reduction classes. So, again, it is difficult to determine which of the changes is most responsible for the health benefit.

A major disadvantage of the Ornish diet is that if you have syndrome X, are diabetic or predisposed to diabetes, or if you tend to have low HDL cholesterol levels or high triglycerides, the diet may lower your HDL (good) cholesterol levels at the same time that it lowers your LDL (bad) cholesterol levels, while also raising your triglycerides. This progression could increase, not decrease, your chances of getting a heart attack.[11] The reason is that when you reduce the amount of fat you eat, the diet typically asks you to replace it with carbohydrates, which requires your pancreas to secrete more insulin to store or metabolize the carbohydrates. This new, higher level of insulin provokes the liver to produce more triglycerides and lower your HDL cholesterol levels, which now fall as your triglycerides go up.

The two basic remedies for this are (1) increasing the amount of exercise you get, which lowers triglycerides and raises HDL, and (2) increasing the unsaturated fat you eat by having a handful of nuts and seeds every day, perhaps some avocado, and using oily salad dressings rather than the low-fat or nonfat varieties. But here we are changing your extremely low fat diet into something that closely resembles the Mediterranean diet (see below). This is exactly what happened to Jacob Gershon (Chapter 8). He tried the Pritikin and the Ornish diets, but on both his triglycerides remained dangerously high and his HDL cholesterol levels dangerously low. Within six weeks of going on the Mediterranean diet, the triglycerides plummeted and the HDL levels shot upward.

If you have no insulin resistance and are not diabetic or prediabetic, or if you do not have low HDL cholesterol or high triglyceride levels, you may do well on an extremely low fat diet. The diet may slow the progression of your coronary artery disease or reverse it, and you may lose weight.

American Heart Association Dietary Guidelines

The American Heart Association (AHA) recommends calorie control and physical activity to achieve and maintain proper weight, and focuses on two entirely different groups of people: healthy persons above the age of two, and those who require a specially designed individual diet, including those with heart disease, high blood pressure, high cholesterol levels, syndrome X, diabetes, or kidney disease.[12]

The guidelines suggest that *healthy persons* look at the big picture, not at individual nutrients, and make healthy choices from each food group in the food pyramid. This would involve whole grains, for example, rather than highly processed carbohydrates, which may raise triglycerides and lower HDL levels. Since many sources of protein also contain fat, the guidelines suggest choosing low-fat sources such as fish, skinned chicken breast, legumes, and low-fat or nonfat dairy, while avoiding red meat or full-fat dairy. The AHA also recommends limiting saturated and trans fats to less than 10 percent of the total calories each day, although persons on weight-loss diets should not replace these kinds of fats with carbohydrates. Those not on weight-loss diets may replace saturated and trans fats with mono- and polyunsaturated fats, as might be found in nuts, seeds, canola oil, olive oil, two servings a week of fatty fish such as salmon, or fish-oil supplements. The recommendation that has received the most attention in the media is that *healthy people* can eat a moderate amount of foods high in cholesterol but low in saturated fat—an egg a day, for example, or one serving of shellfish each day. The AHA also recommends a glass of wine each day, but no more than that, and persons with high blood pressure and certain other conditions should not drink even that much.[13] It is important, however, to consult one's own physician before following this recommendation.

With regard to those for whom this book was written (persons with heart disease, high blood pressure, high cholesterol levels, or diabetes), the AHA recognizes that no single diet will be suitable for everyone, and suggests that each individual consult both medical and nutrition professionals in order to design an appropriate diet.

The reason for this suggestion is that different persons have different dietary needs. The AHA recommends, for example, that persons with high LDL cholesterol levels, syndrome X, or diabetes limit their daily intake of saturated fat to less than 7 percent of calories, and their daily intake of cholesterol to less than 200 mg. But persons with syndrome X or diabetes should also increase the amount of fiber they eat, while persons with high blood pressure or who are in heart failure should restrict their salt intake—in some cases severely. Most people find it difficult to balance these different considerations, which is why professional help is always a good idea.

With the exception of Helen L'Amoreaux, Verne Peters, Jacob Gershon, and Jerry Fox, all of the contributors to this volume try to follow the AHA recommendations.

The Reaven Diet

Gerald Reaven has discovered that eating both carbohydrates and protein makes blood insulin levels go up.[14] Therefore, unlike diets that treat diabetes or the Reaven syndrome by replacing carbohydrates in the diet with proteins, the Reaven diet replaces some of the carbohydrates with unsaturated fats. These fats do not make the blood levels of insulin go up, whereas proteins do, and making blood insulin levels rise is extremely disadvantageous for people with the Reaven syndrome.

In persons with type 2 diabetes, the pancreas is already making all the insulin it can, so eating more protein has no effect on insulin levels and increases glucose levels. If type 2 diabetics eat too much protein or carbohydrate, blood glucose levels will rise; and continuously high blood glucose levels can damage the arteries directly.

The most important feature of the Reaven diet is that it limits carbohydrate intake to 45 percent of total calories. Protein is limited to 15 percent, and the remaining 40 percent of calories are derived from fat. The diet allows fish, poultry, vegetables, fruits, and whole grains, together with unsaturated fats such as nuts, peanut butter, and oily salad dressings. Alcohol in moderation is allowed daily and, because the diet includes only 500 milligrams of calcium per day, those following the diet require daily calcium supplements. The American Diabetic Association recommends the Reaven diet for persons with syndrome X or diabetes, and Shaman Pharmaceuticals, South San Francisco, California, manufactures a dietary supplement formulated by Dr. Reaven called the SynX Bar.

Mediterranean Diets

The Mediterranean diets are those of countries bordering the Mediterranean Sea (Crete, Italy, Greece, southern France, and Spain), all of which have very low rates of heart disease.[15]

Like the extremely low fat diets, the Mediterranean diets are plant based; unlike them, these diets derive 35 to 40 percent of calories from fat, though nearly all will be unsaturated fat from sources such as nuts, seeds, olive oil, and avocado.

The two myths about Mediterranean diets are that they are vegetarian and that they are based on olive oil. As described below, there is much more to these diets than just olive oil. And although these are not vegetarian diets, like all plant-based diets they are rich in vegetables, whole grains, and legumes, as well as foods rich in unsaturated fats and fruits indigenous to the region, such as figs. Unlike a vegetarian regime, however, these diets are flavored with meat.

Typical Finnish and American diets contain a great deal of meat, as well as other sources of saturated fats such as whole milk and cheese. As nutritionists try to figure out exactly what is causing the high rates of heart disease in Finland and the United States, as opposed to the very low rates in countries such as Crete, many questions arise. Are those high rates, for example, the result of the large amount of saturated fats eaten in Finland and the United States, or do foods with those fats displace whole grains and legumes? Does the risk or benefit from a given diet derive from what you eat—or from what you don't eat? Every decision to eat one item is a decision not to eat something else. Nutrition becomes very complex, and none of us know all the answers.

In addition, consider the substantial cultural differences between, say, Crete and the United States or Finland. The Cretan culture requires physical activity (tending flocks, walking), and exercise is known to reduce heart disease. Siestas in the middle of the day are common, and a thirty-minute nap at noon every day has been associated with reducing the chances of having a heart attack.[16]

But there are some signals. Further support for the efficacy of the Mediterranean diet has come from a study in Lyon, France.[17] People who had had heart attacks were divided into two groups; half were on a conventional French diet, the other half on a Mediterranean diet. After four years, those on the Mediterranean diet had 70 percent fewer heart attacks than the control group.

The big advantage of Mediterranean diets, from the patient's point of view, is that they are easy to follow. Fats taste good—we all like them—and the higher fat content of these diets makes them more palatable.

A concern with regard to adding more unsaturated fat to the diet is calories. If the unsaturated fat doesn't replace other calories, then you will be taking in more daily calories, and will eventually gain weight, which will counteract the potential benefits. However, most individuals who change the *type* of calories in their diet typically do so in such a way that the *total* number of calories remains the same (for example, adding a handful of nuts and seeds to the diet, but forgoing a typical evening cookie or bowl of ice cream on the same day).

So if you have high triglycerides and low HDL cholesterol levels, if you have insulin resistance, or if you have diabetes or prediabetes, the Mediterranean diet is preferable to the extremely low fat diets. Similarly, if you find the Ornish-type diets too extreme, if you would rather make smaller changes in your diet and lifestyle, then the Mediterranean diet could be for you. It has two features that protect against heart disease: it is plant based, and it is low in saturated fats.

High-protein Diets

The Atkins and Sears diets have one feature in common: both derive a relatively high proportion of their calories from protein.[18] Atkins first promoted his diet roughly thirty years ago. There are now a number of new high-protein diets, developed after the Atkins and Sears diets. Examples include Protein Power, the Carbohydrate Addict's Diet, and Sugar Busters.[19] But the Atkins and Sears diets differ in major ways. The Sears diet is low fat, low in saturated fats, and moderate in monounsaturated fats, whereas the Atkins diet is high fat (50 percent) and high in saturated fats (about 25 percent) as well as cholesterol (about 880 mg/day).

These diets may have important short-term benefits for obesity. Many people who have had a hard time losing weight find them more helpful than other popular diet plans they have tried—and once the weight is lost, it is easier to take a brisk walk or a bike ride, both of which help to maintain weight loss.

In actuality, these diets have not been studied thoroughly, and there is little scientific information on which to base conclusions. Simplistically, most scientists consider them to be "fad diets," and there is little incentive to study them. Why put energy into researching a diet plan that is likely to be outdated and forgotten by the time the results are collected and published?

All this may be changing. The U.S. Department of Agriculture and the National Institutes of Health have both cited the need to address the discrepancy between the growing popularity of these diets and the lack of scientific evidence as to their potential benefits and risks. It will take several years or longer before meaningful conclusions can be drawn, but the process seems to be under way.

Until then, we do understand that people are more easily satiated on high-protein diets, so they just eat less.[20] Weight loss, remember, has nothing to do with the source of the calories people consume—it depends solely on the *number* of calories. If people are losing weight, they are eating less.[21]

Obesity is a huge problem in the United States, as elsewhere; it is directly linked to heart disease, high blood pressure, syndrome X, and diabetes. So losing weight is really advantageous. If you lose weight on the Atkins or Sears diet—great! However, a key question that remains unanswered is whether people who have lost weight on these high-protein, low-carbohydrate diets are able to keep the weight off. It is long-term loss that counts, and diets have proven to be woefully disappointing in this regard. If these popular diets turn out to be successful in keeping weight under control for several years (and longer) rather than several months, they will have made a substantial health contribution. But that has yet to be demonstrated.

Actively losing weight improves insulin sensitivity. A person with syndrome X or diabetes, for example, will improve as long as that person is losing weight. But if a person with syndrome X who is on a Sears diet does not lose weight, or stops losing weight, insulin sensitivity decreases and insulin secretion increases. Both carbohydrates and proteins increase insulin secretion, and the Sears diet derives 70 percent of its calories from these sources (30 percent from protein, 40 percent from carbohydrates).[22]

In addition, as long as a person is actively losing weight, eating saturated fat does not raise LDL levels. But if someone does not lose weight, or stops losing weight, LDL levels rise—and those LDL levels are an important factor in determining whether that person will have a heart attack.[23] Unfortunately, the Atkins and Protein Power diets derive about 25 percent of their calories from saturated fats.

Finally, from the standpoint of population studies, we have data with regard to low-fat diets in Japan, and the Mediterranean-type diets in Crete and in similar countries; but only Australian Aborigines and Alaskan Eskimos have taken 30 percent of their calories or more from protein over the last few millennia.[24] As discussed earlier, the liver has to detoxify the ammonia generated by the extra nitrogen from these diets, and the kidneys, similarly, must excrete much larger amounts of urea.

These processes tax both organs. However, a recent short-term study has shown that high-protein diets have no adverse effects on kidney function. Whether or not there are adverse effects on the liver, especially after many decades, is not yet known. Finally, ammonia leeches calcium from the bones, causing a four-fold greater risk of breaking a hip in elderly women who eat a lot of meat.[25]

Much of the protein in the Atkins and Protein Power diets comes from meat, which contains methionine. But when people with heterozygous homocysteinemia eat meat, the methionine raises the level in their bloodstream of an amino acid called homocysteine.[26] This substance injures the cells that line the arteries and stimulates the growth of smooth muscle in the walls of those arteries, thereby narrowing the channel through which the blood must flow. High homocysteine levels also increase blood clotting, which can, of course, cause a heart attack or stroke.

Since about 20 percent of people with heart attacks have heterozygous homocysteinemia, and since those with high homocysteine levels have a heart attack level three times higher over a five-year period than those with lower levels, it has been suggested that high homocysteine levels may rival high LDL levels as a major cause of death in the United States and in other industrialized countries. Based on these findings, persons with heterozygous homocysteinemia should not eat much meat, a warning that is once again consistent with the promotion of plant-based diets.

Both the Protein Power and Atkins diets use whole grains and legumes as condiments, substituting proteins for carbohydrates in those foods. But rice is a staple in Asia, as are beans in Latin America, regions where heart attack rates have been low for a very long time.

In conclusion, there have been *no* long-term population studies and *no* long-term controlled studies of the effects of these high-protein diets.[27]

Atkins and Sears have promoted what is now known as the carbohydrate scare. As people in the United States and elsewhere have cut back on fat, their weight, oddly enough, has increased. Atkins and Sears say that it is not wise to cut back on fat and increase carbohydrates. But in our effort to cut back on fat, with what exactly do we replace it?

Let us say you intend to buy a bagel with cream cheese—but you know that cream cheese has a lot of saturated fat, so you have your bagel plain. Yet fat is satiating; you are still hungry, so you have another plain bagel. It is likely that two plain bagels have far more calories than a single bagel with cream cheese. True, you had less saturated fat, but your calories are up.

In an interesting study, researchers gave a group of people yogurt in the early morning. Half the group received nonfat or low-fat yogurt, the other half regular yogurt. The researchers were very explicit with each person about which kind they were getting. What they did not tell their subjects, though, was that they had adjusted the portion sizes so that everyone got the same number of calories. They recorded exactly what each person ate for the rest of the day. All those who had low-fat or nonfat yogurt ate more during the rest of the day than did the people who got regular yogurt.[28]

There are two possible explanations: The first is that the people who were eating regular yogurt were more easily satiated and felt more full; the second is that those on low-fat or nonfat yogurt felt that they had eaten healthily in the morning and were therefore free to eat more later.

The study highlights the fact that people on low-fat diets can ingest an unexpected number of calories and gain weight. The same people might eat only a single cookie, for instance, if they know that it is high in fat, but might eat a whole box of nonfat cookies. The latter, of course, are much higher in calories than the single high-fat cookie.

Another area where this problem arises is in the increasing consumption of soda pop, especially among young people. People think these drinks are healthy because they contain no fat, but they are sugary and high in calories. Besides, the sizes of the cups of soda you can get keep increasing—from a standard 12-ounce (360 ml) cup with about 180 calories, to a 24-ounce (720 ml) cup with about 360 calories, to a 36-ounce (1,080 ml) cup with about 540 calories; now you can even get 72-ounce (2,160 ml) cups, with about 1,080 calories. Clearly, the general population has misinterpreted the low-fat message, thinking that if something is low in fat or nonfat, they can eat (or drink) as much as they want.

Another reason for the increasing obesity in the United States and elsewhere has nothing to do with low-fat diets. Statistics show that the number of people eating out in restaurants increased substantially in the 1990s. Restaurants typically serve foods very high in fat, and in recent years both the size of the serving plates and the amount of food being served has increased. People feel they must finish what is on their plates, so the combination leads to a considerable gain in weight.

Our best current information about what to eat emphasizes predominantly vegetables, whole grains, and legumes as part of a plant-based diet, which would include tofu, soybeans, nuts, seeds, avocados, and oily salad dressings as reasonable options for sources of unsaturated fat.

Medical Foods

The term *medical foods* refers to specific foods that are used to treat a particular disease or condition. Before a manufacturer can call anything a medical food, approval must be obtained from the Food and Drug Administration (FDA), which looks for scientific evidence for the claim that a particular food does what it claims to do. Medical foods are available for the treatment of kidney, liver, and blood-vessel disease, as well as diabetes, burns, and a host of other diseases and conditions.

The development of the first medical foods for heart attack patients was based on the work of three Americans—Robert

Furchgott, Ferid Murad, and Louis Ignarro—who won the 1998 Nobel Prize in Medicine or Physiology for their work.

Essentially, their work showed that an amino acid called L-arginine improves the function of the cells that line the inside of the arteries, which then produce nitric oxide, the most potent substance the body can make for dilating arteries. Numerous studies have shown that elderly people, people with atherosclerosis, and people with risk factors for heart disease produce too little nitric oxide. To get enough L-arginine to counteract this condition, they would have to eat huge amounts of tofu, soybeans, pine nuts, or peanuts—so much that in the process they would get far too many calories and far too much fat. The answer was L-arginine pills; but at least twelve a day would be needed.[29]

To address this problem, John Cooke and his colleagues at Stanford University decided to provide the necessary amount of L-arginine in a candy bar, now called the Heartbar®. It is produced by the company they founded, Cooke Pharma. Each Heartbar® contains not only 3 grams of L-arginine, but also plant estrogens, 250 milligrams of vitamin C, and 200 international units of vitamin E as antioxidants, as well as a large amount of fiber. (For conflict of interest purposes, I must note that I have recently worked with Dr. Cooke.)

Cooke and his group studied patients with intermittent claudication (pain in the legs during walking) due to atherosclerosis in the arteries of the legs. Half the patients in this study were given Heartbar®, the other half a candy bar without L-arginine. The physicians measured with ultrasound the diameter of the arteries in the legs, how far the patient could walk without pain, and the levels of cholesterol and LDL cholesterol in the blood before and after taking two bars daily for two weeks.

In patients on the Heartbar®, the arteries dilated significantly, they walked much farther without pain, and their total cholesterol and LDL cholesterol levels fell significantly. When these data were presented to the FDA, the agency approved the Heartbar® for people with angina, intermittent claudication, diabetes, high cholesterol, and high blood pressure. Both Jacob Gershon (Chapter 8) and Sonny Adams (Chapter 10) were advised to eat two bars a day.

The Heartbar® is no panacea. It includes only a limited number of major nutrients and has been shown to affect only some of the risk factors and symptoms for heart disease. After all, eating a Heartbar® after a hamburger and ice cream would not benefit you. So if you have had a Heartbar®, you have to ask also what did you therefore not eat? Skipping a meal because you have eaten a Heartbar® is not advisable. Drinking two new low-calorie Heartbar® orange flavored drinks a day adds 80 calories to your daily intake.

Nutrition and Heterozygous Homocysteinemia

As discussed above, some people have elevated levels in the bloodstream of an amino acid called homocysteine, which is a risk factor for coronary artery disease. Although three vitamins (folic acid, B_6, and B_{12}) can lower these levels, folic acid (or folate) has proven to be the most effective. The best sources of folate in the diet are beans and green leafy vegetables. Here is yet another example supporting the benefits of a plant-based diet that has to do with factors other than low saturated fat and cholesterol.

In this particular case, mention must be made of the potential benefits of obtaining folate from dietary supplements or fortified foods as opposed to beans and greens. It is known that the folate found in foods is present as a relatively large and complex molecule, a *polyglutamated* folate. In contrast, the folate found in both dietary supplements and fortified foods is present as a smaller molecule, a *monoglutamated* folate. The simpler, smaller molecule is more easily absorbed and therefore more available to your body than the folate from beans and greens. This is not to say that beans and greens are ineffective at lowering homocysteine; it is known that individuals with higher intakes of beans and greens have lower homocysteine levels than those with lower intakes. But it is likely that folate from supplements or fortified foods are even *more* effective at lowering homocysteine levels than folate from beans and greens. Our group completed a study examining this issue and found, in fact, that folate-containing supplements and folate-fortified foods were more effective in lowering homocysteine concentrations than a diet that focused on foods naturally rich in folate (beans, greens, oranges, and orange juice). These data have not yet been published, but are consistent with a study that recently reported a similar advantage of supplements and fortified foods over foods naturally rich in folate.[30]

Phytochemicals

There is yet another reason to consider a plant-based diet, and that is the presence of phytochemicals. These plant chemicals are neither vitamins nor minerals, and supply no calories. They may have benefits for heart disease and diabetes, although this has yet to be proven.[31] Researchers have identified about four thousand phytochemicals, but have studied only about 150. Important examples include isoflavonoids and phytoestrogens from soy, allylic sulfides in garlic, and flavonoids in apples, onions, and tea.[32]

As a simple science lesson, let's say you would like to prove that a certain phytochemical has a beneficial effect. You notice that a certain population has a high rate of heart disease, and another has a low rate. You also notice that these two populations eat different foods.

You work hard for ten years, and finally you isolate a molecule in the food supply of the population with a low rate of heart disease. Maybe that accounts for the difference. Suppose that the molecule in question is the allylic sulfide in garlic.[33] It could be an antioxidant (which disposes of the cell-damaging free radicals in the body, the by-products of the processing of oxygen). You have some evidence too which suggests that it affects the synthesis of cholesterol in the liver.

Once you have isolated allylic acid as something that may be beneficial, you face the huge challenge of making sure whether it is the specific chemical in garlic that helps with heart disease. You find a population with high blood cholesterol levels and give half of them allylic sulfide pills for eight weeks, the other half a placebo, in order to check the effect on total blood cholesterol levels.

But here you face a further problem. What dose should you give? You might give the equivalent of three cloves of garlic a day (which is a lot of garlic!) or one clove a day. Let's say you choose three cloves. At the end of the experiment you find that garlic has made no apparent difference at all. You are about to submit your results for publication when you read an article which shows that when you take allylic sulfide or garlic in an oily form or a tablet, it may have become inactivated by the time it is consumed and absorbed in the body.[34] (This is, by the way, an actual example.)

You would still like to determine the effects of garlic on the body—and, in fact, most people eat garlic, not garlic pills. Hardly anyone eats raw garlic: it is something you cook with. So you think about serving garlic on white French bread smothered in butter (garlic bread); but in this case, if garlic did have any benefits, they would vanish under a load of saturated fat and cholesterol.

You decide to serve the garlic in a stir-fry, or with whole-wheat pasta and vegetables. Now, even if the cholesterol levels come down, you are eating plant-based foods, so all you can say is that the mixture is beneficial. You still do not know what, if anything, is special about garlic.

People eat foods, not nutrients. This is part of the reason why nutrition is so complex. The sum of what a person, or an entire culture, decides to eat is a phenomenon that affects the body as a whole, and deciding which particular part of the total intake is beneficial or not beneficial can get very difficult.

Let us suppose now that you find some other phytochemical that, taken in tablet form, does lower blood cholesterol levels.

This does not necessarily prove that it prevents heart disease; proving that would mean giving a large group of people the tablets in question or a placebo for ten years, and you would have to follow both groups to see how many heart attacks occur in each group. Even then, you would not know if a different dose would have had different effects, or if that particular phytochemical prevents diseases other than heart disease. (To date there have been no ten-year studies on any phytochemical.) So after twenty years of hard work, you have shed only a partial, flickering light on the virtues of that particular phytochemical.

Antioxidants

Antioxidants, for the reasons suggested above, are vital for good health. They probably protect against heart disease, cancer, and a host of other diseases related to nutrition. Animal products—meat, chicken, fish, cheese, milk, and butter—contain *no* antioxidants.

Vitamin E, which occurs alongside unsaturated fats in avocados, nuts, seeds, and salad-dressing oils, was at one time a promising antioxidant. Unfortunately, a recent large study published in the *New England Journal of Medicine* shows that vitamin E supplements do not prevent heart attacks.[35]

Vitamin C, which appears in citrus fruits, guavas, broccoli, tomatoes, strawberries, and kiwis, is another powerful antioxidant. A new preliminary study, however, indicates that large doses of vitamin C may lead to potential problems.[36] Investigators at the University of California, Los Angeles, compared the thickness of the walls of the carotid arteries in people who took more than 480 milligrams a day of vitamin C in tablet form, to those in people who obtained vitamin C from the foods they ate, or who took a daily multivitamin supplement that did not contain more than 480 milligrams of vitamin C.

The result was unexpected. The carotid arteries were almost three times thicker in those taking large doses of vitamin C, compared to those who took took less. And what occurs in the carotid arteries reflects what happens in arteries all over the body.

A five-hundred-page report produced by the Institute of Medicine, a private nonprofit group that advises the United States government, emphasizes that most American get enough antioxidant vitamins from their food. The report concludes that insufficient evidence exists to support claims that large doses of antioxidants can prevent chronic diseases or otherwise improve health.[37]

Many phytochemicals seem promising as antioxidants, especially the carotenoids, including beta-carotene, lutein, and zeaxanthin. They occur in carrots, sweet potatoes, papaya, mangoes, apricots, pumpkin, spinach, peppers, and tomatoes. (Tomatoes also contain lycopene, a carotenoid that may reduce the risk of prostate cancer and heart disease.)

Beta-carotene is an outstanding example of what can go wrong when scientists find an interesting nutritional compound in people with low rates of heart disease. A number of studies initially showed that people with high beta-carotene levels in their blood had less heart disease, and less cancer, than those with lower levels. So the pharmaceutical industry manufactured beta-carotene pills in great numbers. At the time, it was not clear whether beta-carotene actually conferred protection, or was simply a marker for a good diet, or was the marker of an individual who had low risk for other reasons. It was just a piece of the puzzle; those early studies could not show whether beta-carotene was or was not responsible for low rates of disease.

Scientists were already conducting trials in which people were given beta-carotene (in pill form) or a placebo. None of these studies showed any benefit from beta-carotene; in fact, three of those studies, on smokers, showed that beta-carotene had an adverse effect. The smokers who took beta-carotene had more cancer, and more heart disease, than those who did not.

The current conclusion is that *if* beta-carotene is good for you, it should be taken in foods rather than in pill form. To obtain any benefits, you may have to rely on beta-carotene in certain foods, which will occur along with other carotenoids. Beta-carotene may act in a synergistic way with the others, but it will take decades to have a complete understanding of whether beta-carotene is effective, and if so, what the effective dose is, and in what combinations with other carotenoids, and against what diseases. In the meantime, get the beta-carotene you need from a plant-based diet, which we know to be safe.

The Big Picture

There is an important lesson here. When advice appears in the newspapers for or against beta-carotene—or oatmeal, or margarine, or alpha linolenic acid, or omega-3 fatty acids, or any other substance found in food—be skeptical and take it with an ounce of tofu (rather than a grain of salt).

To avoid confusion, remember the big picture.[38] Scrutinize what cultures with low rates of heart disease have eaten for thousands of years. You will discover that all had plant-based diets that are, depending on the region, rich in various combinations of whole grains, legumes, nuts, seeds, avocados, soybeans, tofu, oils with unsaturated fats, antioxidants, and phytochemicals.

These cuisines will be nutritious as well as healthy; often they are colorful and aromatic and contain a variety of spices. There are now a number of cookbooks with recipes for plant-based diets; you can have a brown rice and bean burrito, as would be typical in Latin American cultures; a stir-fry, typical of Asian cuisines; or hummus and tabouli, typical of Middle Eastern cuisines. The foods required for these diets are easy to produce and to harvest and do not spoil as readily as animal foods. They are really extremely practical.

A recent fifteen-year study involving forty-two thousand women found that women who selected foods that fit the new United States dietary guidelines had a 30 percent lower risk of dying from any cause than those who ate the lowest-quality diet. Women who ate the highest-quality diet were 40 percent less likely to die of cancer, 33 percent less likely to die of heart disease, and 42 percent less likely to die of stroke than women who ate the lowest-quality diet.[39] In addition, a prospective study of 44,875 healthy men followed for eight years found that men who ate red meat, eggs, butter, high-fat dairy products and refined grains had significantly more heart attacks than those who ate vegetables, fruit, chicken breast, low-fat dairy products and whole grain products.[40]

We now have a wide choice of diets; you should select one that suits you and your particular medical condition. Keep in mind that the best diet is going to be one that you can maintain over the long haul, day after day, year after year—a diet for life (temporally, and literally). At this time, putting the pieces of the puzzle together (and admitting that many remain to be found), the best message I can offer is to choose:

- A PLANT-BASED DIET
- FROM A VARIETY OF FOODS
- THAT YOU FIND APPEALING, AND PRACTICAL.

CHAPTER 14

Testing and Treatment

Francis H. Koch

Coronary artery disease is the most common form of heart disease in the industrialized world, and it is what most people mean when they speak of "heart disease."[1] Let us look at the anatomy of the heart, the symptoms of coronary artery disease, and the tests used to assess it, before discussing treatment.

The Four Components of the Heart

The first component is the heart muscle, which performs the heart's primary function—to pump oxygenated blood throughout the body.

The second component is the coronary arteries, which supply oxygen to the heart muscle. The heart, like any other muscle, requires a blood supply. Three major coronary arteries supply the heart musculature: the left coronary artery divides into the left anterior descending artery, which carries blood to the front of both ventricles, and the circumflex artery, which supplies the back and lateral wall of the heart; the right coronary artery supplies the right ventricle and part of the undersurface and back of the left ventricle.

These three main arteries then divide into smaller, branching arteries. At birth, all of us have nice clean arterial "pipes." As we age, fatty deposits known as rust develop, which we call hardening of the arteries, arteriosclerosis, or coronary artery disease. When this occurs, the pipes narrow. This process occurs to some degree in all of us. Sixty percent of men 60 years old have some hardening of the arteries. Some people develop symptoms when their arteries narrow; others, however, do not.

The third component of the heart consists of the four chambers in which the blood is received and then pumped to the rest of the body, together with the four valves that regulate blood flow through these chambers. The right atrium is essentially a receptacle, which receives blood as it returns from the rest of the body. From the right atrium the blood is delivered to the right ventricle and then pumped to the lungs, where excess carbon dioxide is released and more oxygen picked up. This rich, oxygenated blood is returned to the left atrium, and from there the blood goes to the left ventricle. The left ventricle is the major pumping chamber of the heart; it sends blood to the rest of the body, as well as to the heart musculature via the coronary arteries.

The oxygenated blood delivers oxygen and other nutrients to various parts of the body. After metabolism has occurred, waste products, including excess carbon dioxide, are returned, via the right atrium, to the heart and lungs.

The heart's valves can become damaged. One valve, called the aortic valve, is located between the left ventricle and the aorta. The aorta is the major artery delivering oxygenated blood to the rest of the body. The mitral valve is situated between the left ventricle and the left atrium. Both of these valves can become scarred and calcified by diseases such as rheumatic fever, or even by the aging process. The other two valves can be affected, but the aortic and mitral valves are most likely to be severely damaged and to require surgery. The artificial valves that the surgeon implants are not perfect replicas of a person's own valves; hence the patient's valves must be significantly damaged before surgery is undertaken.

The remaining component of the heart is its "wiring system." Special tissues in the heart act as pacemakers and tell the heart when and how to beat. "Wires" travel from this special tissue, conducting electrical impulses throughout the heart muscle that make the atria and ventricles contract and the heart beat. Problems can occur within this electrical system. The heart may beat erratically, producing extra heartbeats or sustained irregular heartbeats. These abnormal beats are called an *arrhythmia.* One type of arrhythmia is atrial fibrillation, which originates in the upper chambers of the heart (the atria) and is common in elderly people. It is often controlled or eliminated with medication. Rarely, a pacemaker or specialized surgical procedures are used to treat this condition.

Ventricular fibrillation, another arrhythmia, causes the ventricles to beat inefficiently and is the major cause of sudden death. Persons who have survived episodes of ventricular fibrillation are often given medication and special defibrillators, surgically placed in the heart, to resuscitate the patient should the arrhythmia recur. The internal defibrillator delivers a small shock that converts a weak, irregular heartbeat to a normal beat. The heart's electrical system may fail and the heart may beat too slowly (example, pulse rate = 30). In this case, an artificial pacemaker can be installed to regulate the heartbeat. Both the defibrillator and the pacemaker are placed surgically with a small incision in the chest wall under modest amounts of anesthesia.

Symptoms

Symptoms of coronary artery disease vary widely. Some people develop angina. The classic description of angina is a sense of tightness, squeezing, or pressure in the chest that occurs with exertion and disappears with rest. In my own experience, this definition is incomplete. Angina can be *any* kind of discomfort that predictably occurs with exertion and then goes away with rest. Though angina occurs most commonly in the chest, the discomfort may be in the jaw, shoulder blades, elbow, or pit of the stomach. It is important to emphasize that the discomfort is often not very painful. The key to the diagnosis is its predictability with exertion and relief with rest. Patients with such symptoms should see a physician promptly.

On occasion, there may be no discomfort whatsoever—but there is an inappropriate shortness of breath or fatigue. Someone with coronary artery disease may have climbed the same flight of stairs many times with no difficulty, then abruptly develop significant problems with breathing at the top or become profoundly fatigued. People with these symptoms should also promptly contact a physician.

Tests

To evaluate angina or chest discomfort, an exercise test is often done. This usually involves walking on a treadmill. As the speed of the treadmill and its incline are increased, any symptoms, as well as the pulse rate, blood pressure, and electrocardiogram (EKG), are monitored. The test provides an objective measure of how much exercise someone can do. If, after twelve minutes on the treadmill, there is no angina and no change in the EKG, the outcome is much more promising than if, for example, angina occurs after two minutes of exercise and definite abnormalities appear on the EKG.

The treadmill test is an inexpensive screening to evaluate chest pain or angina. Sometimes the results are equivocal or an extra degree of accuracy is warranted. One of the more sophisticated exercise tests involves the injection of radioactive isotopes into a vein, which defines the portion of the heart muscle receiving inadequate blood flow during exercise. This is called an exercise thallium test.[2] Another technique evaluates the actual beating of the heart muscle just before and immediately after exercise by using painless ultrasound technology (an exercise echocardiogram). This is the same ultrasound technology that obstetricians use to evaluate a developing fetus in the mother's uterus. For patients who cannot exercise, the heart can be stressed by medications that cause the arteries to dilate or the heart to beat rapidly, after which the blood flow to the heart muscle is analyzed by either radioactive or ultrasound methods. Two medications often used to stimulate the heart in this fashion are dipyridamole or dobutamine.

It is possible to obtain specialized X-ray pictures of the amount of calcium present in the coronary arteries (CT scan of the heart). If no calcium is present, one can safely assume that, at worst, only minimal coronary artery disease exists. As more calcium is detected, the amount of coronary artery disease increases. Patients with abnormal calcium scores usually require a functional evaluation, often with one of the exercise tests described above.

The EKG measures electrical activity in the heart. It can become abnormal if the blood supply to the heart is inadequate. Patients with angina at low levels of exercise and with EKG changes often have severe narrowing of the coronary arteries and are at increased risk for a coronary event, such as worsening angina, a heart attack, or sudden death. Conversely, if someone can do a great deal of exercise with little or no angina, and the EKG shows no changes when the heart is beating rapidly, the prognosis is much more favorable.

The exercise test is not without its limitations. For example, it is more accurate in diagnosing coronary artery disease in men than in women—although even in women it is a cost-effective *screening* for coronary artery disease. Although the information obtained from the EKG during the test is less accurate for women than for men, the other data the test generates are equally useful for both genders. The presence or absence of angina, arrhythmias, whether the pulse and blood pressure are normal, and how much exercise a patient can do are all factors that go into the global assessment of each patient's cardiac condition.[3]

The exercise test is not an infallible predictor of future cardiac events, because small areas of narrowing in the coronary artery will not impede blood flow enough to cause angina or EKG changes. Unfortunately, it is these small plaques that often become unstable and rupture, causing a blood clot to form rapidly and acutely block an artery.[4] This process—the rupture of the plaque and subsequent clotting of the artery—can cause complete blockage of an artery, leading to a heart attack or a dangerously irregular heartbeat (ventricular fibrillation) causing sudden death. A heart attack occurs when an inadequate supply of oxygenated blood is delivered to a portion of the heart muscle. This dead heart muscle eventually turns into scar tissue and no longer beats normally.

If a patient is seen soon after a heart attack, clotbusters (what physicians call thrombolytics) are used. These agents help break up the clot that caused the heart attack. Thrombolytics given soon after a heart attack save lives. In patients who have survived a heart attack, medications called beta-blockers and ACE inhibitors have been demonstrated to prolong life.

As is evident from the above statements, a major dilemma facing physicians is that minimal coronary artery disease can abruptly lead to severe blockage of an artery, causing a heart attack or death. We have no adequate way to predict which patients with mild disease are going to have such a bleak outcome.

On the other hand, if the tests described above suggest the presence of severe coronary artery disease, the physician may perform an angiogram, particularly if he or she suspects that the patient is a candidate for a procedure to increase the blood flow to the heart.

An angiogram involves placing a tiny tube called a catheter into the origins of the coronary arteries (often through an artery in the groin). Through the catheter a special dye is injected that outlines on a type of X-ray film the degree of narrowing in the vessels. Depending on the results of the angiogram, one of two procedures can follow. The first, which may be done as soon as the angiogram is completed, is an *angioplasty.* A special balloon-tipped catheter is passed into narrowed areas of the coronary artery. The balloon is then inflated, which squashes the intruding plaque back against the wall of the artery, dilating the inside of the artery and improving blood flow to the heart muscle.

During this procedure, the cardiologist may also place a special metal scaffolding, called a stent, into the narrowed area.

The major limitation of angioplasty is the artery's reaction to the disruption of the plaque. In this reaction, known as restenosis, scar tissue is formed. The scarring can be very extensive and cause at least as much narrowing of the vessel as was there prior to the procedure. Restenosis can occur in 10 to 50 percent of cases, depending on a number of factors. Currently there is no satisfactory method to predict or prevent restenosis. In general, the bigger the lumen of the artery after the procedure, the lower the chance of restenosis. ("Bigger is better.")

The angiogram helps to determine whether angioplasty or a coronary bypass operation is indicated. When a bypass is done via open-heart surgery, an artery or vein from elsewhere in the body is used to reroute the blood supply past the blocked artery or arteries. If this procedure is recommended, the cardiologist will refer the patient to a cardiovascular surgeon.

Patients who have some damage to their heart muscle and all three vessels significantly blocked have improved survival rates after a bypass operation compared to patients treated only with medications.

The Foundation Approach

I personally approach everyone with coronary artery disease with what I call the "foundation approach." A foundation of *medical management* is the basis for *all* treatment of coronary artery disease. On top of this foundation, specialized procedures such as angioplasty or bypass surgery may be added. These procedures are done "in addition to" medical therapy, not "to replace" medical therapy. The patient who has had procedures must continue to be diligent in following a medical regimen.

The first principle of the foundation approach is that there are actions patients must take to help themselves.

The second principle is that there are actions the physician must take to help the patient.

As these statements imply, patient and physician have a partnership, and it is vital that both understand their roles and work together toward the same goal.

The patient's responsibility is to make the lifestyle changes discussed in Chapters 1, 13, and 16. The more steps the patient takes to boost coronary health (diet, exercise, smoking cessation), the less medication and fewer procedures specialists will need to provide. It should be comforting to patients to know that they have some control over their prognosis.

The physician's first responsibility is to make sure each patient is fully aware of and understands the risk factors for heart disease, and the importance of trying to modify them in the interest of better cardiac health. The second responsibility is to provide medications that will modify some of the risk factors, and help to control the symptoms of heart disease.

Medications to Modify Risk Factors

To Lower Cholesterol

Bile-acid sequestrants, niacin, fibrates, and statin drugs all lower cholesterol. When an initial angiogram of an untreated patient and one done several years later are compared, it is evident that arteriosclerosis can progress over time. Cholesterol-lowering drugs, however, can slow the rate of progression.[5] Patients taking these medications develop fewer fatty deposits in their arteries. In addition, nearly all angiographic studies have shown that in a small percentage of patients taking these medications, coronary artery disease may even regress to some degree.

Similar angiographic data are present for some patients on a very strict low-fat diet without specific lipid-lowering drugs. All studies involving lipid-lowering medications advise the patient to be on a low-fat diet.

Niacin is an effective lipid-lowering drug. It reduces the

chance of a second heart attack and prolongs the lives of patients who have had an initial heart attack.

Fibrate-type medications (for example, gemfibrizol or fenofibrate), similarly, can reduce the chances of a heart attack.

The most widely prescribed cholesterol-lowering drugs are the statins. Most studies showing the beneficial effects of cholesterol-lowering drugs on the heart and blood vessels were performed with statins. Some of the statin drugs reduce the chances of having a heart attack or of needing a bypass operation or angioplasty. A recent study suggests that, for patients with modest coronary artery disease, taking a statin-type medication is as beneficial as angioplasty. Other studies have demonstrated that taking some of the statin drugs can actually prolong life. In addition to these cardiac benefits, statin drugs also reduce the incidence of strokes by 20 to 30 percent.

The statin drugs do more than just lower cholesterol.[6] Whereas cholesterol levels can be ascertained, not all processes in the body are easily measured. Various studies in humans and animals have shown, for example, that statin drugs tend to relax the arterial walls and help prevent them from contracting and going into spasm. Other studies have shown that they prevent fatty plaques in the walls of the arteries from rupturing. Additional research has suggested that the statin drugs reduce inflammation, which can be associated with a tendency for plaques to rupture. We cannot routinely measure how reactive a patient's arteries are, or whether the plaque in an artery is unstable. As noted previously, it is the rupture of this plaque that causes most of the acute problems of coronary artery disease. In the opinion of many investigators, such processes (vascular reactivity/spasm, plaque rupture, and inflammation) can be favorably modified by statin drugs.[7]

The statin drugs and bile-acid resins work very well in lowering LDL cholesterol levels, but are less effective at lowering triglycerides and elevating HDL cholesterol. By contrast, niacin and the fibrate group of drugs are more effective at this latter task. Niacin is probably the single best agent for elevating HDL and lowering triglyceride levels.

If physicians cannot get HDL, LDL, and triglycerides to a desirable level in their patients, they may use combinations of these agents to do so: niacin may be added to a statin drug, for example, or niacin, statin drugs, and a bile-acid sequestrant may all be tried, in various combinations, to see what works best in a specific patient. When this is done, there is often a synergistic effect; the combination of drugs is more effective than any single drug by itself. However, as the dose of statin-type drugs is increased, it produces a proportionally smaller reduction in cholesterol levels. For example, if a 20-milligram dose produces a 20 percent reduction in LDL cholesterol levels, a 40-milligram dose might yield only a further 10 percent reduction.

All cholesterol-lowering drugs have side effects:

- Bile-acid sequestrants look and taste like sand, and usually cause constipation. However, newer forms of bile-acid sequestrants are now available in pill form. Since they are not absorbed in the bloodstream, there are no systemic side effects; hence these are very safe agents. Very rarely, they can cause exacerbation of asthma.
- Niacin often causes itching and flushing of the skin, but many people can minimize this side effect if they start with a low initial dose and gradually increase the dose over time. Low-dosage aspirin taken with niacin will often reduce the flush. Niacin typically starts to have a beneficial effect when the dose reaches about 1,500 milligrams per day.
- Niacin, statin drugs, and fibrates can cause abnormalities of blood tests related to liver function and muscle enzymes. Yet if only one of these drugs is being taken, the chance of such a side effect is about 1 percent. It is uncommon for anyone to develop symptoms related to abnormal blood-test results. Very rarely, sustained-release types of niacin can cause severe liver inflammation (hepatitis), which can result in the need for liver transplant and/or death. Also

very rarely, patients may develop myalgias (a sense of the muscles being sore, tender, or stiff), when the muscle enzyme levels are abnormal. All cholesterol-lowering drugs can cause upset stomach or constipation, but these symptoms too are rare.

To Control Blood Pressure

Serious consideration should be given to controlling high blood pressure with agents such as diuretics, beta-blockers, and ACE-inhibitor–type medications, since they can help prevent future cardiac events. It should not be forgotten that blood pressure medications definitely reduce the chances of a stroke.

To Control Diabetes

Diabetes can be controlled by using diet, pills, or insulin—and doing so may help prevent future cardiac events. Favorably modifying high blood pressure and cholesterol levels improves a diabetic patient's cardiac prognosis.

Medications to Control Symptoms of Heart Disease

Angina is a frequent manifestation of coronary artery disease, caused by an imbalance of the available oxygen supply and the oxygen demand of the heart. Beta and calcium channel blocking drugs can help modify that imbalance by slowing the heart rate and lowering the blood pressure, so that the heart does not demand as much oxygen for a given amount of work. Beta-blockers can also prolong survival in someone who has had a prior heart attack.

Nitroglycerine is a crucial medication. It relieves angina promptly by dilating the coronary arteries. (It also dilates other arteries and veins in the body, helping to lower the blood pressure and therefore making the heart work less.) Patients who experience angina should take nitroglycerine whenever the angina does not promptly disappear. They should also take nitro-glycerine prophylactically (that is, if they know they will be in a situation that might provoke an anginal attack, such as sexual activity, walking up several flights of stairs, or a stressful argument). Long-acting nitroglycerine preparations (isosorbidini-trate) can be very effective in preventing anginal episodes.

Many physicians tell their patients to abide by the "three by five" rule. If angina has not subsided after taking one nitroglyc-erine tablet, take a second within five minutes. If angina is still present five minutes later, take a third pill. If the angina persists after fifteen minutes and three pills, go immediately to the hospital and notify your physician that you are doing so.

Aspirin is a great medication for patients with vascular disease. It is inexpensive, reduces the chances of a second heart attack, and has very few side effects (upset stomach) or risks (bleeding into the bowel or brain). Multiple studies have shown that, for patients with vascular disease, the benefits of aspirin far outweigh its risks.

Angiotensin is produced in many parts of the body and contributes to the constriction of blood vessels. ACE inhibitors lessen this effect; they dilate the blood vessels and help lower blood pressure. ACE inhibitors also prolong life in those who have had damage to their heart muscle.[8] A recent study of an ACE inhibitor called Ramipril® has shown that it can prevent heart attacks and strokes in patients who are at risk for the complications of vascular disease.[9]

Another of the physician's responsibilities is to determine whether patients are indeed modifying their risk factors and taking their medications. To do this, the physician will ask patients what risk factors they are modifying, and which medications they are taking. A compliance study done to evaluate patients taking statin drugs showed that many stopped their medications within one year.

The physician will also monitor the results of various tests to see if goals are being achieved. A standard goal, for example, is to have a cholesterol less than 200, a cholesterol/HDL ratio of three to one or lower, and an LDL level of less than 100 mg/dL (2.6 mmol/L) and a triglyceride level less than 150 mg/dL. These recommendations are based on the recent National Cholesterol Education Panel III guidelines, published in 2001.[10]

For diabetic patients, many physicians attempt to reduce hemoglobin A1c (Hgb A1c) to as close to normal as possible (less than 7 mg/dL). For hypertensive patients, they will attempt to get the blood pressure below 140/90. If a patient is diabetic, the goal is often less than 135/85.

Unfortunately, despite making appropriate lifestyle modifications and taking medications faithfully, people can still develop progressive coronary symptoms. Angina, for example, can become incapacitating, which often means that at least one of the major coronary arteries is significantly narrowed. When symptoms become this severe, another stage of treatment becomes necessary, and a physician will often recommend an angiogram, to determine if an operative procedure is warranted. If the angiogram shows that only one of the major coronary arteries is significantly blocked, the physician will usually recommend an angioplasty and stenting (PTCA—Percutaneous Transluminal Coronary Angioplasty).[11]

If severe symptoms and significant disease are present in two of the three coronary arteries, the degree of technical difficulty in attempting an angioplasty and the wishes of the patient will dictate the next step, which could be either angioplasty or a bypass procedure.

However, if all three coronary arteries have significant disease, the physician will usually recommend a bypass procedure.[12] For patients who have some damage to their heart and significant blockage of all three major vessels, a bypass operation can not only help alleviate symptoms, but also prolong the patient's life.

Like any surgical procedure, a cardiac bypass operation has a downside. Unlike angioplasty (with or without stent placement), after which the patient can usually leave the hospital the next day, a bypass procedure involves opening the chest and a patient can expect to spend five to seven days in the hospital afterward. Very rarely, there are complications from the general anesthesia. Angioplasty is done under local anesthesia and avoids the risk of general anesthesia.

During the bypass operation, the patient is usually placed on a heart/lung machine. The heart is stopped, and the machine takes over the function of the heart and lungs. Complications such as a stroke are occasionally associated with this machine. Pneumonia and kidney damage are potential but unusual complications of heart surgery. Arrhythmias, such as atrial fibrillation, are not uncommon, but usually disappear by the time the patient is discharged.

The risk becomes greater the older the patient, the more severe the coronary artery disease, and the worse the preoperative heart, lung, and kidney function. Diabetes adds a further hazard to any operative procedure. In most patients the risk of death, heart attack, stroke, or other serious complications is low. Continued medical therapy, angioplasty, and bypass surgery *all* have potential risks and benefits, and these must be weighed by the patient and the physician before any decision is made about the preferred treatment option. Continued medical management, for example, may be more risky than a bypass operation.

The left anterior descending artery is often the most favorable one for bypass; the internal thoracic (also known as the internal mammary) artery can be attached to it. Postoperative arteriosclerosis rarely develops in this artery-to-artery bypass procedure. Follow-up angiograms usually reveal that the arterial grafts are patent and functioning well five, ten, and even fifteen years after the surgery.

Arteriosclerosis develops at a much faster rate, however, when the surgeon uses veins, typically from the leg, to bypass diseased arteries. About 50 percent of patients with vein bypass grafts will develop a cardiac event within ten years. This cardiac event can be a serious complication (a heart attack or sudden death, or the need for another bypass procedure or angioplasty) or a minor complication (the return of angina). In 10 to 15 percent of patients, angina will recur within one year of a bypass operation.

One theory as to why arteriosclerosis occurs so quickly with vein surgery is that veins are not accustomed to the high blood pressure to which arteries are routinely subjected, and they therefore develop accelerated disease. However, it is always puzzling to a heart surgeon during a second operation to see one vein graft that is very diseased and, inches away, another vein graft that is just as old but looks pristine.

When the surgeon can graft one artery to another (typically the left internal mammary artery to the left anterior descending), the operation is successful in about 95 percent of cases. When it is not successful, it is usually because of a technical problem, perhaps difficulty in suturing the arteries together.

Depending on the patient's anatomy, surgeons can sometimes do two arterial bypass procedures during one operation, utilizing both internal mammary arteries or one internal mammary artery and the patient's radial artery (the artery taken from the wrist area and used by the physician to assess a patient's pulse).

A number of new bypass procedures have been developed. One involves doing the bypass on a beating heart, thereby eliminating the heart/lung machine, the hypothesis being that avoiding the heart/lung machine will reduce the chance of a stroke. Skillful surgeons can do this procedure on multiple arteries; many, however, prefer to work only on the left anterior descending artery when the heart is in motion.

Other surgeons have developed a procedure that requires only a small incision in the chest, as opposed to cutting through the entire breastbone, which has been the routine bypass procedures for years.

A third new approach involves special equipment and small incisions in the chest wall to both see and work on the heart.[13] A slender, flexible optical instrument known as an endoscope is utilized to examine the inner part of the chest while, at the same time, the surgeon performs the surgery through very small incisions in the chest, using specialized instruments.

Surgeons believe that these new approaches reduce the length of time that it is necessary to stay in the hospital, the severity of pain after the procedure, and complications such as arrhythmias after the surgery. As yet, however, there is no proof that these novel approaches lead to a more prolonged life span or fewer heart attacks than does the standard procedure.

In general, women do slightly less well than men after angioplasty, stenting, or bypass procedures. One theory suggests that because a woman's arteries are smaller than a man's, either the inside cannot be dilated as well with angioplasty and stenting, or if bypass surgery is done, too little blood flows to the small artery from the graft. Further, women tend to develop varicose veins during pregnancy, after which those veins may be less suitable for bypass procedures.

Having a bypass procedure (or angioplasty) is not like having an appendix removed. Once the appendix is gone, there is no longer a possibility of appendicitis. A bypass procedure or angioplasty merely buys more time. Therefore, no matter what "high-tech" vascular procedure is done, it is important to return to medical management of the risk factors for coronary artery disease.

Conclusion

The emphasis of the foundation approach is on the patient and the physician working together to modify those factors that can be changed, to help slow the progression of coronary artery disease and forestall the need for high-tech interventions. When a high-tech intervention is performed, medical management remains crucial to avoid the necessity for another high-tech procedure. Patients have a great deal of control over their own outcomes, and by vigorously modifying their risk factors they can improve those outcomes.

CHAPTER 15

An Introduction to Cardiac Rehabilitation Programs

Kathleen Berra

Cardiac rehabilitation in the United States has undergone an incredibly rich and energizing thirty years. In the late 1960s you could count on the fingers of one hand the number of cardiac rehabilitation programs in this country. But Gary Fry, an especially enthusiastic and visionary cardiologist at the Palo Alto Medical Foundation in California, knew instinctively that there had to be something better than building more and more coronary care units for victims of heart attacks. His vision, his passion, was to keep people out of coronary care units, out of hospitals, and to keep them well.

Little was then known of the value of reducing risk factors for heart disease, although the dangers of smoking, high blood pressure, diabetes, and high cholesterol were understood. The benefit of reducing those factors was supported by some data, but far less was known about the importance of high cholesterol, of chronic stress, of being overweight, of not exercising, and of not eating properly.

Nevertheless, in 1970 Dr. Fry decided to establish a freestanding cardiac rehabilitation program, in the community, away from the hospital setting. Distance was the key: he wanted to stay away from the all-too-familiar illness environment, and almost physically establish that heart attack patients would be learning about wellness in an environment free from all the associations of illness. It was at this point that I became involved in his dream. Our goal was quite simple: to provide health education, medically supervised physical activity, and risk reduction programs that would reduce death and disability from heart attack and stroke.

My own background had been in coronary care, and independently I had come to care deeply about helping patients stay well after a heart attack, and about improving the quality of their lives. I was committed to the health of the patients, of their families, and of the community.

The rest, quite literally, is history. In the last thirty years, enormous amounts of data have been accumulated that strongly support the benefits of cardiac rehabilitation. Our knowledge of how to modify risk factors for recurrent heart attack and stroke, and of the efficacy and safety of reducing those risk factors, has increased enormously. The news is unequivocal: a huge number of patients now benefit from belonging to cardiac rehabilitation programs, and today there are thousands of these programs in the United States alone. Most hospitals that treat patients with heart disease and stroke either have their own on-site program or participate in a large program in the community, such as the one here in Palo Alto.

In order to develop what came to be a huge number of programs dedicated to cardiac rehabilitation, and to educate and encourage professionals to pursue cardiac rehabilitation as a career, the American Association of Cardiovascular and Pulmonary Rehabilitation (AACVPR) was established in 1986. I am pleased to say that I was a founding member.

This new organization was important because many disciplines needed to be represented in a single organization. Existing institutions, though helpful, were already very large, which made it difficult for them to embrace this new syncratic movement.

In the beginning, the American College of Sports Medicine

was extremely influential, because of its vast knowledge about exercise, clearly a key component of rehabilitation. The American Heart Association was also strongly supportive from the start. But we needed to reach in other directions; during my term as the fledgling organization's second president, our goal was to increase the membership and to attract the interest and participation of the many specialists who would be needed —nutritionists, exercise physiologists, nurses, physicians, psychologists, and psychiatrists. The efforts of all these specialists would be to ensure that patients in cardiac rehabilitation received the greatest possible benefit. These early efforts proved to be a great success and within a few years the AACVPR had more than three thousand members.

Nor was this all. The association helped to inspire similar groups throughout the world. The first was a very strong organization in Canada, which was soon followed by other groups in Europe and throughout the world.

The United States cannot take credit for the initial development of cardiac rehabilitation programs as such. From the late 1940s on, spas in West Germany began to offer patients who had had a heart attack programs in stress management, exercise, and nutrition. Guests at these spas could stay as long as six weeks.

Building on this early start, Germany continues to stay in the forefront of cardiac rehabilitation. Germany was joined by Sweden, where coronary artery disease was rampant, and the two countries are today seen as leaders in the field. The United States has learned a great deal from both.

More recently still, excellent programs have begun in France, Spain, Italy, Russia, Poland, Israel, the United Kingdom, Ireland, Australia, South Africa, China, Indonesia, the Philippines, and Japan. Cardiac rehabilitation has achieved enormous international importance.

All of the programs are similar in one major way: they strive to reduce the risk factors for recurrent heart attack and stroke. Data from these programs have provided overwhelming evidence that they are effective in achieving this goal.

Although heart disease remains the major cause of death and disability for both men and women in the United States, living with coronary artery disease is much easier than it was thirty years ago because of the lifestyle changes people make after developing heart disease. In addition, significant advances have been realized in the pharmacological treatments for atherosclerosis and coronary risk factors. Further, the public understands that getting to the hospital as soon as possible after developing symptoms of a heart attack provides the very best chance of a favorable outcome. Many technologies, including angioplasty, stenting procedures, clotbuster therapies, and advances in bypass surgery have helped to ensure better outcomes for persons with coronary artery disease.

Another important advance has been the integration of pulmonary rehabilitation programs with cardiovascular programs. Pulmonary programs provide benefits similar to those I have enumerated to persons with diseases of the lungs such as emphysema and asthma. Many individuals have both cardiac and pulmonary disease and therefore profit from the expertise of the pulmonary and cardiac professionals who manage these programs. The future promises to bring greater integration of a variety of rehabilitation programs to make the best use of professional expertise and program space.

In 1995 the AACVPR published the first evidenced-based clinical guidelines for cardiac rehabilitation, under the aegis of the United States Agency for Healthcare Policy and Research. These guidelines showed clear-cut evidence that cardiac rehabilitation works.[1] Subsequently, the World Health Organization and many rehabilitation associations in countries around the world have published their own rehabilitation guidelines.

The ideal cardiac rehabilitation program places heavy emphasis on lifestyle changes. The skills of the specialists in the program are geared toward helping patients make and maintain the lifestyle changes they need: smoking cessation, lowering of cholesterol, weight reduction, exercise, stress management, and good nutrition.

Besides inquiring about lifestyle, there are other fundamental questions one should ask about rehabilitation programs:

- What are the facilities like? Is there space for stationary exercise equipment, relaxation, upper-body training? Are swimming facilities available?
- Who supervises the program?
- Is there a medical advisory committee?
- Are there specially trained nurses, exercise specialists, and nutritionists? Is the program associated with the AACVPR?
- Are the exercises individually designed, depending on a person's specific condition?
- What types of risk reduction programs are offered?
- Are the nutrition programs directed and taught by a skilled nutritionist?
- Is there a weight control program?
- Is a stress management course offered? Are individual and group stress management programs available?
- Can one get help to stop smoking?
- Can spouses participate, and is there a support group for spouses and families?
- How long does the program last? Is there an option for long-term participation?

In conclusion, you should know that in joining a cardiac rehabilitation program, you will acquire new ways to manage your risk factors for heart disease and stroke. You will learn how to exercise safely and how to monitor your own signs and symptoms. You will know when to call your doctor and when you do not need to worry. You will learn ways to manage your medications, the benefits of those medications, how to evaluate their effectiveness, and how to take them properly—all in an effort to provide you with the best possible results. You and your family will benefit from your improved sense of self-confidence, improved physical capacity, and greater sense of well-being.

Apart from these benefits, you will undoubtedly find that there are some surprising benefits from your regular attendance at your rehabilitation program, including a growing camaraderie and support system. Even regular attendance itself has benefit—a lot of people in rehabilitation say to themselves, "While I'm in the program, at least I know I'll be exercising regularly and making the lifestyle changes I need to make."

There is probably a cardiac rehabilitation program somewhere near you. Whether you stay for six weeks, six years, or the rest of your life will depend on your own needs and what is available in your community. But do not hesitate! Joining a cardiac rehabilitation program is fun and rewarding in many ways. To find a program in your community, call the AACVPR at (609) 831-6989 or call the local office of the American Heart Association or a similar organization.

CHAPTER 16

Cardiac Rehabilitation in Action

Donna Louie, Nancy Houston Miller, and Robin Wedell

If you had a heart attack in the United States in the 1950s, you would have had to stay in the hospital for six to eight weeks and not move out of your bed. During the next six months, you would have been allowed very little physical activity.

If you had a heart attack in the 1960s, you would have been much more fortunate, because it was then that the first programs were developed in the United States to promote appropriate exercise as part of your recovery.

If you had your heart attack in the 1990s, though, you would have been the beneficiary of some truly amazing changes. If your heart attack had been treated with clotbusting drugs, if you had had an angioplasty (in which arterial narrowing is dilated with a balloon), or if a stent (a tubular metallic mesh that expands to keep the artery open) had been inserted after the angioplasty, you would have discovered that your rehabilitation began the day after the heart attack.

This is truly an enormous change. Whereas exercise was once thought to be harmful, it is now seen as integral to the recovery process.

Western Europeans can be proud that virtually 100 percent of persons with heart attacks join a cardiac rehabilitation program afterward. The record in the United States at present is not as favorable. In various parts of the country where cardiac rehabilitation programs are available, only 11 to 38 percent of heart attack patients enroll.[1]

Cardiac rehabilitation programs all over the world are very similar, with only minor variations, so our description of a typical program in the United States also applies to other places in the world where such programs are available.

Initial Steps

When you join a cardiac rehabilitation program, you assume responsibility for your own health and wellness by managing what has now become a chronic (rather than an acute) disease. The main objectives of the program will be to find out what risk factors you had for heart attack, and why you had the attack; to develop goals that are mutually agreed on by you, the program staff, and your doctor; and to establish a mutually acceptable plan to achieve those goals.

Reading about and understanding your risk factors is just one aspect of your road to recovery. Joining a cardiac rehabilitation program takes you a step farther by helping you put lifestyle changes into practice. The staff's contribution is to change your behavior. Your entry into a program is the beginning of a positive, supportive experience in health maintenance and lifestyle changes.

The cardiac rehabilitation program tries, essentially, to reduce the likelihood that your heart disease will progress. In order to do that, it is necessary to look at a large number of factors that need to be addressed, and to devise appropriate strategies to achieve the following goals:[2]

- Cessation of smoking
- Total cholesterol less than 200 mg/dL (5.2 mmol/L)
- Low-density lipoprotein cholesterol (LDL) level less than 100 mg/dL (2.6 mmol/L)

- High-density lipoprotein cholesterol (HDL) level greater than 40 mg/dL (1.0 mml/L)
- Triglyceride level less than 150 mg/dL (3.9 mmol/L)
- Blood pressure level below 135/85 mm Hg
- Best possible control of diabetes (fasting blood glucose 110 mg/dL or lower, and hemoglobin A1c less than 7.0)
- Regular exercise three to five times per week in the target heart range, as defined by the treadmill test (which establishes what your target or safe heart rate should be)
- Maintenance of a healthy body weight and body-fat percentage (body mass index or BMI less than 25)
- Management of stress.

The values for total, LDL, and HDL cholesterol, and for triglycerides, for people who have had a heart attack are based on current guidelines published by the National Cholesterol Education Panel III, published in 2001. These guidelines apply to people with clinical coronary artery disease, symptomatic carotid artery disease, peripheral arterial disease, abdominal aortic aneurysm or diabetes. Blood pressure guidelines are based on the current recommendation of the Joint National Commission on Hypertension VI. However, it is felt that a lower blood pressure, in the range of 120/70 mm Hg, is much better. Guidelines for the normal values of fasting blood glucose and the hemoglobin A1c test are those of the American Diabetic Association in 1999.

The staff in the best possible cardiac rehabilitation program will include (at a minimum) a physician, nurses, an exercise physiologist, a registered dietitian, and a psychologist.

Your actual treatment plan involves a team consisting of you, your doctor, and the cardiac rehabilitation staff. If you would like to enter a cardiac rehabilitation program, you must be referred by your doctor, as all such programs must be medically supervised. The program will require your medical records. The staff then does a detailed initial evaluation, which has three components: reviewing your medical history, identifying your learning needs, and establishing goals for reducing your risk factors for a heart attack.

Reviewing Your Medical History

The reason everyone with heart disease needs to be evaluated before beginning a cardiac rehabilitation program is that there are medical conditions that might make it dangerous for you to participate, or prevent your participation, or require changes in the kinds of exercises you do. Your medical records are invaluable for this purpose, as is a personal interview, to make sure that your exercise prescription is both appropriate and safe.

Identifying Your Learning Needs

For your part, you will need to understand exactly what is going on with you medically, what caused your coronary artery disease, and precisely which risk factors contribute to your heart problem. You will then set goals to reduce your risk of further problems and learn how to monitor yourself during exercise.

Here is what you will need to do:

- Identify angina if you are experiencing it, and start treating it immediately.
- Use the Borg scale[3] to evaluate how much you are exerting yourself.
- Recognize subtle signs that your heart disease may be worsening, such as unusual shortness of breath, increasing fatigue, or a decreasing ability to exercise as much.
- Understand the meaning and the importance of the target heart rate guidelines.
- Stop exercising during illness, or if you develop more angina, or under certain other conditions.
- Use all available resources to help enhance your lifestyle changes.
- Stay motivated to make lifestyle changes.

• If you have a history of congestive heart failure, learn to check your weight daily; a sudden increase in weight could indicate that you are retaining water, which could worsen your heart failure.

The staff will provide you with written information to enable you and your family to understand these goals and challenges. You will also be given an analysis sheet that details your personal risk factors, and other written information that explains your personal guidelines for safe exercises.

Establishing Your Risk Factor Goals

The program staff will review all known risk factors with you and determine which you need to change. With their help, you will then set your own personal goals, which are mutually agreed upon and which can prevent you from developing further heart problems. It is extremely important that you be actively involved in establishing these goals, because your ultimate success depends on your motivation and your confidence that you can achieve them.

In addition, your cardiac rehabilitation program will be offering a large number of other experiences, which may include individual counseling, group classes, lending libraries, written materials, tours, and demonstrations.

The Role of Exercise

Exercise is the cornerstone of all cardiac rehabilitation programs. A sedentary lifestyle is a major risk factor for developing heart disease, comparable in seriousness to the other principal risk factors.

Exercise decreases your risk of developing future heart problems and, if you reduce all your other risk factors at the same time, you may live longer.

How does exercise do this?

- It lowers your blood pressure.
- It increases your HDL (good) cholesterol level.
- It lowers your triglycerides.
- It helps you lose weight and maintain your weight loss.
- It helps you to manage diabetes, as it decreases your insulin resistance and improves glucose tolerance.
- It decreases blood clotting, leading to a lower risk of heart attack and stroke.
- It makes the inner lining of your arteries healthier and more efficient.
- It reduces depression and anxiety and enhances feelings of well-being.

Exercise for persons with heart disease is not without risk, especially if you have not been properly evaluated. For your safety, the staff will work out specific guidelines about how much you can exercise and how to do so safely. If you follow these guidelines, exercise can be both healthful and fun. Remember also that the staff will keep in close contact with you, helping you to evaluate any new symptoms that may occur while you are exercising. They will also request a treadmill exercise test to ensure the safety of your exercise prescription.

You will sometimes hear people say about exercise, "Just take it easy," or conversely, "Don't baby yourself." These kinds of offhand remarks can be misleading and dangerous, and they are nothing like what your professional rehabilitation staff will say to you.

Your professional rehabilitation staff will begin by thoroughly assessing your medical history, your personal beliefs, your behavioral characteristics, the medicines you are taking, your age, and your work situation. Each is equally important, and all are factored into your exercise prescription.

The Best Exercise Program

The amount of exercise needed to reduce your risk of a heart attack is much less than would be needed to keep physically

fit. If you have never exercised at all, you can significantly reduce your chances of a heart attack by walking for as little as
ten minutes three times a day. But you should not aim simply at
reducing your risk of a heart attack; the idea is to keep fit, especially if you are older, because in doing so you will reduce your
risk of falling and injuring yourself, and allow yourself to keep
up with your daily activities (shopping, for instance). The fact
that Helen L'Amoreaux (Chapter 5) exercised in a cardiac rehabilitation program for twenty years eventually saved her life—
in a most unusual way. She was in a near-fatal auto accident, but
survived solely because she was in almost unbelievable physical shape.

An appropriate exercise program allows you to select activities you enjoy and that you will do often enough, long enough,
and to a degree that will keep you fit.

In organizing their thinking about exercise, cardiac rehabilitation programs pay special attention to the Frequency, Intensity, Time, and Type (FITT) of exercise.

Frequency = at least three to five times a week
Intensity = at your target heart rate
Time = thirty minutes on each occasion
Type = the exercises you enjoy.

Researchers on exercise normally quantify the amount of exercise you have done in terms of the total calories burned. Many
exercise machines (such as exercycles) have monitors that help
you calculate the number of calories you are expending.

Current data show that the least number of calories you
should burn to protect yourself against heart disease is 700 a
week. Most cardiac rehabilitation programs will try to get you
to burn about 1,000 calories per week. To get in the best shape,
and to give yourself the best protection from coronary artery
disease, you need to burn 2,100 calories a week, or 300 a day. If
you have coronary artery disease and are still working, this goal
can be very challenging.

A comprehensive cardiac rehabilitation program employs

four components in your exercise prescription: exercises that improve aerobic capacity, muscular endurance and strength, coordination, and flexibility. Paying attention to all these aspects will enable you to continue functioning optimally for many years.

Your exercise prescription should consider not only your functional capacity, but other factors that may limit the kinds of exercises you do, such as problems with bones, joints, and tendons.

In a cardiac rehabilitation program, exercise classes are normally supervised by registered nurses and exercise physiologists. Registered nurses have experience working in coronary care units (CCUs) and are able to read electrocardiograms. They can immediately recognize when the heart muscle is not getting enough blood, or when irregular heart rhythms are occurring. In addition, all nurses in the program are trained and certified in advanced life support techniques. A defibrillator and a crash cart, with oxygen and all the appropriate medicines, is available so that on those rare occasions when you might need help, you can be treated immediately and appropriately. (In some programs your heart rhythm may actually be monitored via telemetry for the first few weeks, with your heart's rhythm visible on a screen.)

Often after a heart attack or bypass surgery, a person may be sensitive to physical symptoms or changes. The medical supervision available in your cardiac rehabilitation program will help sort this out. The nurses, who will know you and your history very well, can assess any new symptoms or changes in symptoms, weight gain, medication changes, and your progress with lifestyle changes. This supervision can be very reassuring, as you will learn more about which symptoms matter and which do not. The nurses, with backup from your doctor if required, can tell you whether your symptoms are significant or trivial; even when your symptoms have significance, the problems often will be caught early enough that they can be dealt with before they become serious.

Finally, nurses and other staff are selected for their empathy and their enthusiasm. These traits can help significantly in persuading you to initiate the lifestyle changes you need to make.

Exercise physiologists or other well-qualified exercise instructors will lead a typical exercise class with ten minutes of cardiovascular warm-up and range-of-motion exercises. You will be asked to take your pulse before and after the warm-up, the goal being to increase your heart rate to near your individual target heart rate. (That rate will have been determined from the exercise stress test taken earlier.) This warm-up phase is critical, which is why it is led by an exercise physiologist or a well-qualified exercise instructor. Warm-up ensures that your heart (as well as the surrounding muscles and tissues) is getting enough oxygen, which lowers the risk of angina and general muscle fatigue.

After the warm-up period, everyone embarks on their own exercise program; typically, an aerobic phase of about thirty minutes follows the warm-up. Each person works with a variety of equipment; some programs may also offer walking exercises or dance or water aerobics.

During this aerobic phase and at any other time during exercise you will be cautioned to report any of the following symptoms immediately, should you have them:

- Chest, arm, jaw, neck, or back discomfort or pressure
- Very rapid or very slow heart rate
- Irregular heartbeats
- Shortness of breath, such that you have difficulty carrying on a conversation with fellow members of your program
- Fatigue or weakness
- Dizziness
- Nausea.

While you exercise, you will learn to take your own pulse, to use a scale to rate your perceived level of exercise,[4] and to check yourself for any relevant symptoms.

This aerobic phase will be followed by a cool-down period,

typically of about fifteen to twenty minutes, which has the following goals:

- To bring your heart rate back to its pretraining level
- To practice stretching so as to increase your flexibility
- "Resistive training," the chief purpose of which is to build muscle mass and increase your strength, which will contribute significantly to your health and independence in years to come.

(Resistive training may involve working with weights or rubber bands or machines with chains and pulleys, to simulate actual weights. In each case the weight or resistance will be geared to what you can handle at that stage of your physical training.)

At the end of your cool-down period, you will measure your pulse rate, which should be close to your rate before exercise. You will have an exercise sheet to document your progress, which will ask you many questions:

- What is your resting pulse rate?
- What is your high pulse for the day?
- What is your rating of your perceived exertion?
- What is your recovery pulse rate?

In addition, if you have any angina during the class, or if you have irregular heartbeats, there will be further questions to answer regarding those developments.

In order to answer these questions, you will need to monitor yourself carefully during exercise. When you first enter a cardiac rehabilitation program, the nurses will teach you how to do this—and, with practice, you can become very proficient. The goal, incidentally, is not simply to detect problems that may require treatment; monitoring yourself teaches you to be comfortable with your own body, to learn what your heart can and cannot do, and to monitor yourself so well that after a time you may be able to guess your heart rate with great accuracy, just by how you feel!

Diet

But cardiac rehabilitation does not end with exercise. Diet too is vitally important to your overall health. Your cardiac rehabilitation program may offer classes, grocery-store tours, cookbook libraries, cooking demonstrations, and recipe exchanges, all in an effort to educate you and to encourage you to think differently about what you eat. Eating a low-fat, high-fiber diet is most effective in reducing one's cholesterol level. The common framework is a diet that is low in saturated fat. Total fat content may vary individually, based on medical history and dietary needs (see Chapter 13).

Cardiac rehabilitation programs help you make dietary changes in a positive, supportive, and educational environment —one in which, for example, you will learn how to read food labels and understand what to eat and why.

Stress

Who doesn't have stress? We all do; but how much stress you have and how you cope with it can have a significant impact on your health.[5]

For heart attack patients, stress and type A behavior might as well be synonymous. Historically, the term "type A behavior" arose because a couple of cardiologists, Doctors Meyer Friedman and Ray Rosenman, were trying to get a grant to study the effects of anger and stress on the heart. The government agency administering the grant said, however, that only psychologists or psychiatrists, not cardiologists, could apply for grants to study anger and stress. Someone at the agency said they could overcome the problem by calling the visible signs of anger and stress type A behavior, which they did—and the grant was forthcoming.

Many people have the impression that stress is a personality trait that must be changed. In fact, it is a behavior pattern, a habitual way one acts or conducts oneself. If you find that you react to issues in your daily life with anger, irritation, aggravation, or impatience, those responses generate stress hormones that can damage your cardiovascular system. You can learn to replace those feelings with healthier responses such as acceptance, high self-esteem, affection, and serenity through a type A modification course. Stress exists in all of our lives, but what creates the most stress in *your* life may be quite different from the triggers in the lives of others. Recent studies on a psychological system called the Enneagram, for example, suggest that people can be grouped according to nine different personality types, each of which reacts differently to stress.[6]

The original cardiologists recorded the physical signs of these characteristics on videotape, so that their work was behavioral rather than an exploration of the personality itself.[7] The physical signs of stress and anger (type A) visible during the videotaped clinical examination included:

- Dark rings around the eyes
- A tic-like drawing-back of the corner of the mouth while speaking
- Rapid tic-like eyebrow lifting
- Rapid (more than forty per minute) eye blinking
- Explosive staccato speech
- Hand waving
- Fist pounding
- Finger wagging at the examiner
- Head nodding during speech
- Interruption of the examiner's speech.

Understanding stress and anger is essential to helping people better manage it. Anything that reduces self-esteem, first of all, causes anger or hostility. The misunderstanding arises because self-esteem is confused with self-confidence. Self-esteem is an internal feeling regarding one's worth, as opposed to self-confidence, in which others receive the impression that a person is confident. People with low self-esteem can exhibit high self-confidence, and it may require experience and expert testing to distinguish between the two.

A second area of confusion involves the relation between the term "workaholic" and stress. Those who have found that workaholics do not have more heart attacks did not know that there are two distinctly different kinds of workaholics—the hardworking person and the hard-driving person. Working hard and long hours does not have to cause stress if someone loves the work and is relaxed doing it. The hard-driving person, on the other hand, has a compulsion to succeed or excel, and is fiercely competitive. He or she works long hours under a great deal of stress, and is much more likely than the hard worker to have a heart attack or other cardiac problems—or another heart attack if the individual has already had one.

There is confusion too about the number of hours worked versus stress. A recent study has shown that working shorter hours does not necessarily prevent heart attacks. This conclusion has unfortunately given rise to the erroneous idea that being a so-called workaholic does not lead to heart attacks. But when people try to cram the same amount of work into fewer hours, the level of stress goes up enormously. In fact, whenever a deadline is imposed, one's stress level almost always rises, and the chances of having a heart attack increase.

Oddly enough, most heart attacks occur in the morning. Part of the reason is that epinephrine levels are highest then, due to natural circadian rhythms—but those higher levels tend to constrict the coronary arteries. That is probably why Jose Ibarra (Chapter 2) and Hans Forsell (Chapter 3) had their heart attacks in the morning. Stress can also play a role, since it too raises epinephrine levels. In the morning if you are late for work, if there are traffic jams, if other drivers are irritating, if you begin to feel enraged—you may be at risk for a heart attack. Becoming angry while driving is dangerous for other reasons as well. Dr. Ricardo Martinez, the former national highway safety administrator, has shown that road rage causes twenty-eight thousand fatalities a year in this country. The solution, clearly, is to rise a little earlier, dress and have breakfast in a relaxed way, leave early enough to allow for delays, and drive in as relaxed a fashion as possible.

Stress and anger can have a number of harmful effects:

- Raise the blood level of epinephrine, which can lead to high blood pressure, spasm of the coronary arteries, an irregular heart rhythm (which can be life threatening), and blood clot formation by blocking the action of aspirin on the blood platelets and thereby increasing the activity of the platelets.
- Raise the blood level of cortisol, which if chronically elevated can lead to type 2 diabetes, which in turn is a risk factor for heart attacks.
- Decrease vagal control (the vagus nerve helps to calm and restore you).
- Cause sludging (rouleaux formation) of the red blood cells after a high-fat meal, which could block the collateral vessels bypassing narrowed coronary arteries.
- Elevate the blood level of LDL cholesterol.
- Elevate the blood level of triglycerides.
- Increase the blood level of homocysteine (see Chapter 13).
- Decrease the ability of the cells forming the inner lining of the arteries to function properly.

Friedman and his colleagues were the first to study the effects of behavior modification in heart attack patients. They found that time urgency can be alleviated via a number of techniques, including replacing certain old beliefs with new ones, changing behavior, and revising daily activities. The new beliefs are that time urgency does not lead to social and economic success and that change is possible, even in covert insecurity, the underlying basis of time urgency. Behavior can be changed by using verbal imagery in daily thought, taking an interest in the lives of others, learning how to be a human *being* rather than a human *doing,* and by becoming more cultured. Daily activities can be revised—by determining which daily activities can safely be dispensed with, and by simple changes like allowing idling time before and after the morning toilet and breakfast, and recognizing that breakfast itself can be a pleasurable event. Minibreaks throughout the day can be effective, as can trying not to get all the work done by a certain time, if doing so causes stress and time urgency. Finally, creating an internal self-monitor can be very helpful.

Anger and hostility too can be treated by developing new beliefs and by changing behavior. New beliefs include reinforcing the fact that hostility is not needed to get by in the world, that it is possible to reduce hostility, and that it is unhealthy to regard other people as ignorant and inept. They include as well that one can live with doubt and uncertainty, and that giving and receiving love are signs of strength, not of weakness. Behavioral changes include developing new ways to give and receive love and to develop understanding, compassion, and forgiveness in dealings with others. They also involve searching for the beauty and the joy in life, stopping the use of obscenity, and monitoring internal hostility levels. Several changes in time urgency and hostility involve the nourishment of a spiritual life, and a richer and deeper spiritual life often accompanies the management and reduction of stress.[8]

Making all these changes is neither easy nor automatic, and requires daily attention. A typical practice exercise might be the following: Walk more slowly and notice your surroundings. This carefully researched drill works on many levels. The slower pace removes the "Urgent" message the body sends to the brain when rushing. And focusing on nature is more relaxing than letting your mind go into a problem-solving mode.

Making these lifestyle changes involves more than simply one's beliefs and actions. Recent research has shown that altering beliefs and behavior can actually rewire the brain, so that this work changes not simply *who* you are, but also *what* you are.

After these kinds of behavior modifications, people see themselves and the world very differently.[9] They become more accepting of themselves and not excessively self-demanding or critical. If they face a difficult situation or a deadline, they encourage themselves by remembering how capable they are and that they have survived demanding people or situations before. They do not berate themselves for their inadequacies or their failures.

They expect and experience a sense of harmony with the people, events, and circumstances in their lives. For this reason they are team players, able to lead or let others lead, and they do not experience a lot of friction, opposition, combativeness, or competition for control in their personal or professional relations.

They notice the good in the people or events surrounding them, and are not preoccupied with what is wrong. They are willing to trust the good in others, and look beyond mistrust, suspicion, wariness, and cynicism.

The external appearance of people who have undergone behavior modification may change. Their posture and movements become more relaxed, their gestures more natural, and their faces in repose more relaxed and friendly. Their voice becomes easy to listen to, and their speech is evenly paced and unhurried. They express real interest in others and listen patiently while others speak.

And those in the presence of persons who have made these changes notice that their mood has become more dependably pleasant and that they are more accepting and interested in others. Jacob Gershon, Verne Peters, and Sonny Adams all reported noticing changes in their behavior that made them more enjoyable to those who were around them. The trivial mistakes and differences in ways of doing things become unimportant; in the face of big mistakes, people take a calm, problem-solving approach, displaying a new and unexpected flexibility. Such persons avoid being overwhelmed by momentary difficulties and match effort to the importance and difficulty of the task, bearing in mind that not every task requires all-out effort. They develop a sense of enjoyment and fulfillment with the process as well as with the outcome of their work.

In the recurrent coronary prevention study, a randomized study involving 862 men and women who had had heart attacks, Friedman and his colleagues were able to demonstrate that if patients underwent appropriate behavior modification, the recurrence rate after four and a half years was 44 percent lower than in a control group that had not undergone behavior modification. Dr. Friedman wanted to continue the study longer, but the National Institutes of Health, which had funded the study, felt that the interim results were so convincing that it would be unethical not to treat the control group. This study was selected as one of the most significant psychopathological studies done in the last thirty years, and in 1993 was given the Upjohn Award of the International Society for Behavioral Medicine. All of this work has been replicated by additional studies that have used the video interview and the diagnostic criteria established by Friedman and his colleagues.

Other investigations have shown that relaxation exercises, biofeedback, and meditation can reduce the chances of a repeat heart attack as much as 40 to 74 percent.[10] You may even find that not until you join a cardiac rehabilitation program do you understand what being relaxed feels like. Only then can you truly learn to differentiate between relaxation and stress.

For these and other reasons, many cardiac rehabilitation programs offer stress reduction and type A behavior modification classes, typically lasting eight weeks to a year. They can generate a very significant reduction in your chances of another heart attack!

Support for Your State of Mind

After a heart attack, bypass surgery, or other revascularization and treatment such as angioplasty or stenting, you are likely to feel anxious and depressed, and as though your body has betrayed you. But there is a vicious circle here: Depression increases your risk of another heart attack, by two- to threefold, and can slow your recovery. Studies show that if you have the support of family and friends, you are less likely to have another heart attack or die.[11]

So how you feel and whether or not you have support can be crucial in preventing heart attacks. This is why, during your initial evaluation, the cardiac rehabilitation nurses will tell you that it is normal to feel frightened and depressed after a heart attack, but that the feeling is normally temporary and may lessen as you progress with your program. If your depression fails to resolve, the nurses will help you seek additional support such as counseling or medications. All cardiac rehabilitation programs encourage you to bring members of your family with you to the initial evaluation. Doing so can give you emotional support at a crucial time, which will strengthen your motivation to achieve your own goals and those of the program.

The camaraderie and support you will derive from the program is paramount and will probably surprise you. Your exercise instructor, for example, is more than just someone who tells you what exercises to do. To be sure, he or she will approach you while you are doing your aerobics and ask how the exercise is going, but that person will engage you in meaningful social interaction as well. In fact, your exercise instructor, like all the staff in your cardiac rehabilitation program, performs a social function that goes beyond what you might expect from your local gym.

Nor is this the only support you can expect to receive. The nurses will also be with you, monitoring your physical condition and chatting, asking how you are doing—talking, really, about anything at all. The point, once again, is to engage and support you in the life you are living.

Another important benefit is the other members of your class. They too will get to know you, and after a few months you will discover that they care about you and that you have made a number of new friends. Very often they will call or visit if you are sick, and they may expand their social lives (as you may expand your own) to include other participants in the program. Jerry Fox (Chapter 12), for example, reported that his best friends—indeed, his only friends—were people he met in a cardiac rehabilitation program. And when, as he lay dying of cancer, these friends visited and comforted him, each helped him to remain calm and peaceful to the very end.

This social and emotional side of cardiac rehabilitation is enormously important and often unexpected. But it does occur, as if miraculously, and will help you recover much faster and more completely than if you try simply to exercise on your own.

Healthy Pleasures

A number of studies have shown that "healthy pleasures" significantly reduce the chances of having a heart attack or other heart procedures, or of having a second heart attack. These healthy pleasures include:[12]

- Thinking optimistically
- Having sex twice or more a week
- Drinking a glass of red wine every day
- Taking a thirty-minute siesta every day
- Having a playful dog or purring cat nearby
- Enjoying a satisfying marriage (divorce, on the other hand, significantly increases the chances of heart attack)
- Touching people while speaking to them
- Indulging in selfless pleasures such as generosity, helping someone in need, altruism (volunteering, for example, on a regular basis), being grateful for all you receive.

If you live in an industrialized country, you are more apt to have a heart attack or other heart problems than if you live in a slower-paced environment. Whether or not you do, your number one priority after a heart attack is to identify the risk factors you can change and set goals to begin making those changes.

A cardiac rehabilitation program can help get you on your feet again and set your plan in motion.

If you live in the United States, it is likely that your physician will enroll you in a cardiac rehabilitation program, enabling you to enjoy all of its benefits. If this does not happen, seek out a program yourself (see Chapter 15).

The challenge for the new millennium, in the United States and elsewhere, is to increase membership in cardiac rehabilitation programs to a level comparable to those in Western Europe, where referral is automatic.

Home-based Rehabilitation

Home-based cardiovascular rehabilitation extends services to those who do not have access to a formal cardiac rehabilitation program. Unfortunately, only 11 to 38 percent of all American patients who have coronary heart disease are able to avail themselves of the services provided through formal rehabilitation programs in hospitals and community settings such as YMCAs or Jewish community centers.[13] Extending the availability of what we know to be the safe elements of exercise and rehabilitation enables a larger proportion of the 14 million Americans who now suffer cardiovascular disease to receive these types of services.

Home-based rehabilitation encompasses the majority of services that are provided in a traditional rehabilitation program. Included are exercise conditioning, risk factor education and counseling, and ensuring that patients receive the appropriate medical therapies known to improve long-term outcomes. Studies of home-based rehabilitation actually began in the mid-1970s, and have included patients who have had a myocardial infarction, coronary artery bypass surgery, and percutaneous coronary angioplasty.[14] In the randomized controlled studies of these populations, outcomes including functional capacity have been comparable to those involving individuals in traditional programs. Most recently, studies suggest that exercise training at home may be suitable for elderly patients, including those with heart failure and even those who have undergone heart transplantation.[15]

Remember, taking appropriate measures to ensure your safety if you are exercising at home is critically important prior to undertaking this form of rehabilitation. If you are graduating from a formal cardiac rehabilitation program or exercising in a home program to begin with, you must have medical clearance, understand methods of monitoring your intensity of exercise, be aware of the signs and symptoms that require medical attention, and receive clearly delineated guidelines that identify the frequency, intensity, time, and type of exercise to be performed (FITT guidelines). Written guidelines that include an exercise prescription are therefore crucial before you begin exercising at home. Moreover, individuals need to be aware of exercises that may improve musculoskeletal conditioning and those that should be avoided (such as heavy isometric exercise).

If you have had a heart attack, most likely you will undergo a treadmill test or other functional tests to clarify the appropriate intensity of exercise for you. If such tests have not been performed, use of the Borg Perceived Exertion and Pain Scales [16] may be a valuable method of monitoring exercise intensity. You may also benefit from the general guideline of using a "resting heart + 20" beats during exercise conditioning, especially if you are not taking beta-blockers to prevent your heart rate from rising significantly.

Some form of surveillance or close monitoring is also relevant to the safety of home exercise training. From the early 1970s on, transtelephonic monitoring has helped to assure patients that they may exercise safely at home. Transtelephonic monitoring from a remote site can detect irregular heartbeats and inadequate oxygen to the heart muscle during exercise training in individuals who may be at slightly greater risk for cardiovascular problems. Such monitoring has also been used to connect people during exercise sessions so that they receive external support, something that is not normally available in a home program. Finally, transtelephonic monitoring has been used to monitor one's compliance with an exercise program. (Another method of surveillance is weekly or even monthly telephone contact by nurses and other rehabilitation staff who are skilled in identifying complications from exercise training and changes in your symptoms.)

One of the best ways to ensure that home exercise training is incorporated into your daily routine is to encourage you to undertake monitoring skills that will help you continue with the exercise program. A daily exercise log in which to record the number of minutes exercised, including any changes in symptoms, can be mailed to personnel overseeing those involved in home rehabilitation programs.

Home-based rehabilitation also encompasses risk factor counseling and education to ensure that you receive appropriate therapies that promote long-term improved outcomes. One way to provide these services is through the use of nursing case management. In a study of patients recovering from a heart attack, DeBusk and colleagues found that patients followed by nurses primarily by telephone as part of a home-based rehabilitation program showed significant improvement in smoking cessation, lipid levels, and functional capacity when compared to those receiving the usual care from their physicians.[17] In this system of care, known as MULTIFIT (Multiple Risk Factor Intervention Trial), nurses manage patients with cardiovascular risk factors and other chronic conditions such as heart failure, diabetes, or hypertension. The twelve-month home-based program offers patients up to four face-to-face clinic visits and 911 telephone contacts for follow-up and surveillance. In addition, patients complete exercise logs, dietary reports, and laboratory requests as needed. The individual face-to-face sessions provide ongoing education and counseling. Average telephone contacts of ten minutes offer support, reinforce education provided through written materials and face-to-face sessions, and enable nurses to suggest problem-solving skills to enhance compliance. Nurses also respond to questions patients may have about their overall recovery and lifestyle changes. While home rehabilitation programs such as MULTIFIT do not offer the psychological group support found in formal rehabilitation programs, support groups in medical centers, the community, and through the Internet may supplement patients' needs for these services.

Notes

1. Heart Attack and You

1. G. Reaven, T. K. Strom, and B. Fox, *Syndrome X: Overcoming the Silent Killer That Can Give You a Heart Attack* (New York: Simon and Schuster, 2000).

2. United States Centers for Disease Control and Prevention Morbidity and Mortality Weekly Report, August 6, 1999.

3. M. M. Lipman and colleagues, "Heart attack: What's your risk?" *Consumer Reports on Health* 11 (April 1999): 1; F. J. Pashkow and colleagues, "Patient, screen thyself," *Cleveland Clinic Heart Advisor* 2 (August 1999): 1; Mayo Clinic, *8 Ways to Lower Your Risk of a Heart Attack* (Rochester, Minnesota: Mayo Clinic Foundation for Medical Education and Research, 1999); D. L. Sprecher and colleagues, *Heart Attack Prevention: Lowering Your Risk for Heart Disease* (Stratford, Connecticut: Torstar Publications, 2000).

4. H. C. Herrmann and colleagues, "What is a lipid profile?" *Heart Watch* 3 (April 1999): 2; F. J. Pashkow and colleagues, "Age is no excuse: Controlling cholesterol is important," *Cleveland Clinic Heart Advisor* 2 (November 1999): 1; F. J. Pashkow and colleagues, "Keeping cholesterol in check: Are you doing all you can?" *Cleveland Clinic Heart Advisor* 2 (October 1999): 1; F. J. Pashkow and colleagues, "How high are your triglycerides and why should you care?" *Cleveland Clinic Heart Advisor* 2 (January 1999): 6; J. S. Alpert, "HDL on the rise," *Health News* 5 (September 10, 1999): 4; S. Margolis and colleagues, "Can cholesterol lowering be too aggressive?" *Johns Hopkins Medical Letter, Health After 50* 11 (August 1999): 3; T. H. Lee and colleagues, "Cholesterol tests: The good, the bad, and what's healthy," *Harvard Health Letter* 25 (November 1999): 6; T. H. Lee and colleagues, "Lowering cholesterol," *Harvard Health Letter* 25 (September 1998): 8.

5. Expert Panel on Detection, Evaluation and Treatment of High Blood Cholesterol in Adults, *Journal of the American Medical Association* 285 (2001): 2486.

6. F. J. Pashkow and colleagues, "Homocysteine: Is it time to be tested? Recommendations are changing," *Cleveland Clinic Heart Advisor* 2 (Septem-

ber 1999): 1; T. H. Lee and colleagues, "Beyond cholesterol: Clusters of risk factors," *Harvard Heart Letter* 9 (October 1998): 3; S. E. Goldfinger and colleagues, "B vitamins and heart disease," *Harvard Health Letter* 23 (October 1998): 8.

7. R. S. Lang, "What to do about the new markers of cardiac risk," *Cleveland Clinic Men's Health Advisor* 2 (March 2000): 6.

8. B. Liebman, "Multiple choice: How to pick a multivitamin," *Nutrition Action* 27 (April 2000): 1.

9. G. Sheps and colleagues, *Mayo Clinic on High Blood Pressure* (Rochester, Minnesota: Mayo Clinic Foundation for Medical Education and Research, 1999); T. H. Lee and colleagues, "Isolated systolic hypertension," *Harvard Heart Letter* 8 (October 1997): 8; T. H. Lee and colleagues, "Changing the tone of blood-pressure controls," *Harvard Heart Letter* 8 (July 1998): 1; T. H. Lee and colleagues, "Hypertension: A need to get pushy," *Harvard Heart Letter* 9 (October 1999): 5; O. K. D. Aaronson, "What's the safest blood pressure?" *Heart Watch* 2 (August 1998): 1.

10. G. Reaven, T. K. Strom, and B. Fox, *Syndrome X: Overcoming the Silent Killer That Can Give You a Heart Attack* (New York: Simon and Schuster, 2000); H. C. Herrmann and colleagues, "Preventing heart disease in people with diabetes," *Heart Watch* 2 (September/October 1998): 1; T. H. Lee and colleagues, "Searching for coronary disease among people with diabetes," *Harvard Heart Letter* 9 (March 1999): 1; D. M. Nathan, *Diabetes* (Boston: Harvard Medical School Health Publication Group, 1999).

11. B. M. Berman and colleagues, "Secrets of successful losers: Losing weight doesn't have to be a losing battle," *Consumer Reports on Health* 12 (January 2000): 1; G. G. Blackburn, "Losing weight: A little goes a long way," *Health News* 5 (November 20, 1999): 1; M. N. Walsh, "Body shape affects heart risk," *Heart Watch* 3 (January 1999): 4.

12. E. Koop, Shape Up America BMI Chart, http://www.shapeup.org/bmi/chart.htm.

13. T. H. Lee and colleagues, "Heartburn can cause real heartache," *Harvard Heart Letter* 6 (August 1996): 7; S. Margolis and colleagues, "When chest pain isn't a sign of a heart attack," *Johns Hopkins Medical Letter, Health After 50* 11 (December 1999): 6; F. J. Pashkow and colleagues, "Is it a heart attack or something else?" *Cleveland Clinic Heart Advisor* 1 (September 1998): 1.

14. R. S. Lang and colleagues, "Puzzling out chest pain: Is it a heart attack? Or something else?" *Cleveland Clinic Men's Health Advisor* 2 (January 2000): 6.

15. T. H. Lee and colleagues, "Medical errors: Patient, protect thyself," *Harvard Health Letter* 25 (February 2000): 3; R. Sandroff and colleagues,

"Avoiding hospital blunders: Knowing the risks and speaking up can help you stay safe," *Consumer Reports on Health* 12 (June 2000): 1; A. S. Brett, "Medical errors: Often preventable, seldom litigated," *Journal Watch* 20 (April 15, 2000): 68.

13. The Complexities of Proper Nutrition

1. G. Reaven, T. K. Strom, and B. Fox, *Syndrome X: Overcoming the Silent Killer That Can Give You a Heart Attack* (New York: Simon and Schuster, 2000); B. Liebman, "Syndrome X, the risks of high insulin," *Nutrition Action Health Letter* 27 (March 2000): 4.

2. Ibid.

3. L. F. Larsen, J. Jesperson, and P. Marckman, "Are olive oil diets anti-thrombolitic? Diets enriched with olive, rapeseed, or sunflower oil affect postprandial factor VII differently," *American Journal of Clinical Nutrition* 70 (December 1999): 976.

4. B. Liebman, "Plants for supper?" *Nutrition Action Healthletter* 23 (October 1996): 10–12.

5. C. Perry and colleagues, "For a whole heart, whole grains," *Tufts University Health and Nutrition Letter* 16 (October 1998): 1.

6. S. E. Goldfinger and colleagues, "The neglected nourishing bean," *Harvard Health Letter* 23 (September 1998): 1.

7. M. Friedman, *Type A Behavior: Its Diagnosis and Treatment* (New York: Plenum, 1996), pp. 10–12.

8. R. Pritikin, *The New Pritikin Program: The Easy and Delicious Way to Shed Fat, Lower Your Cholesterol and Stay Fit* (New York: Simon and Schuster, 1990).

9. D. Ornish, *Dean Ornish's Program for Reversing Heart Disease: The Only System Scientifically Proven to Reverse Heart Disease without Drugs or Surgery* (New York: Ballantine, 1990).

10. J. A. McDougall, *The McDougall Program for a Healing Heart: A Life-saving Approach to Preventing and Treating Heart Disease* (New York: Plume, 1998).

11. Reaven, Strom, and Fox, *Syndrome X;* Liebman, "Syndrome X"; C. Perry and colleagues, "Should *you* be eating *more* fat and *fewer* carbohydrates? If you have a condition called syndrome X, too many carbohydrates could prove bad for your heart," *Tufts University Health and Nutrition Letter* 16 (February 1999): 1; T. H. Lee and associates, "Triglycerides: Bad actor or innocent bystander?" *Harvard Health Letter* 21 (May 1996): 2–6.

12. AHA dietary guidelines: Revision 2000. http://circ.ahajournals.org/cgi/content/full/102/18/2284.

13. K. Conger, "Hats off to alcohol: A researcher's fanciful vision of hats dangling on hat racks within our cells explains how alcohol protects against heart disease," *Stanford Medicine* (Fall 2000): 21.

14. Reaven, Stromp, and Fox, *Syndrome X*.

15. T. H. Lee and colleagues, "Sail your way to a healthy heart. The Mediterranean diet," *Harvard Heart Letter* 10 (October 1999): 1; S. Margen and colleagues, "Just what exactly is the Mediterranean diet?" *University of California, Berkeley, Wellness Letter* 15 (April 1999): 3; S. Margen and colleagues, "Remarkable heart benefits from canola oil," *University of California, Berkeley, Wellness Letter* 15 (May 1999): 1; J. E. Brody, "Savory diet that's good for heart? Let's eat," *New York Times,* section D6, March 23, 1999; C. Perry and colleagues, "Yes, but *which* Mediterranean diet?" *Tufts University Health and Nutrition Letter* 17 (April 1999): 1.

16. D. Trichopoulos and colleagues, "Does a siesta protect from coronary heart disease?" *Lancet* 2 (August 1987): 269.

17. See note 15.

18. B. Sears, *Mastering the Zone: The Next Step in Achieving Super Health and Permanent Fatlessness* (New York: Harper Collins, 1997); R. C. Atkins, *Dr. Atkins' New Diet Revolution: The Amazing No-hunger Weight-loss Plan That Has Helped Millions Lose Weight and Keep It Off* (New York: Avon, 1997).

19. M. R. Eades and M. D. Eades, *Protein Power* (New York: Bantam, 1999); B. Liebman, "Diet versus diet," *Nutrition Action* 23 (May 2000): 9.

20. R. D. Sheller and colleagues, "High-protein, low-carb diets: Are they right for you?" *Mayo Clinic Health Letter* 18 (July 2000): 4.

21. S. Margen and colleagues, "Eat fat, get thin?" *University of California, Berkeley, Wellness Letter* 16 (April 2000): 1.

22. Reaven, Strom, and Fox, *Syndrome X*.

23. Sheller et al., "High-protein, low-carb diets."

24. Eades and Eades, *Protein Power*.

25. D. E. Sellmeyer and colleagues, "A high ratio of animal to vegetable protein increases the rate of bone loss and the risk of fracture in postmenopausal women," *American Journal of Clinical Nutrition* 73 (January 2001): 188.

26. R. S. Lang and colleagues, "Is it the new cholesterol? What you should know about homocysteine," *Cleveland Clinic Men's Health Advisor* 2 (June 2000): 4; J. E. Brody, "Health sleuths assess homocysteine as culprit," *New York Times,* section D1, June 13, 2000.

27. M. Jacobson, "Popular diets: Untested," *Nutrition Action* 27 (May 2000): 2.

28. D. J. Shide and B. J. Rolls. "Information about the fat content of pre-loads influences energy intake in healthy women," *Journal of the American Dietetic Association* 95 (1995): 993.

29. G. S. Frances and colleagues, "Why cardiologists are just saying NO: Scientists eager to identify nitric oxide's role in heart disease," *Cleveland Clinic Heart Advisor* 2 (October 1999): 3.

30. L. J. Riddell and colleagues, "Dietary strategies for lowering homo-cysteine concentrations," *American Journal of Clinical Nutrition* 71 (2000): 1448.

31. S. Margen and colleagues, "Beyond vitamins: The new nutrition revolution," *University of California, Berkeley, Wellness Letter* 15 (April 1999): bonus insert.

32. S. Margen and colleagues, "Green, black, and red: The tea-total evidence," *University of California, Berkeley, Wellness Letter* 16 (March 2000): 1.

33. T. H. Lee and colleagues, "Garlic: Can it keep your blood vessels young?" *Harvard Heart Letter* 8 (March 1998): 6; T. H. Lee and colleagues, "Garlic oil: No impact on lipids," *Harvard Heart Letter* 9 (September 1998): 6.

34. Lee et al., "Garlic oil."

35. Heart outcomes prevention evaluation study investigators, "Vitamin E supplementation and cardiovascular events in high-risk patients," *New England Journal of Medicine* 342 (2000): 154.

36. N. S. N. Gershoff and colleagues, "New questions about the safety of vitamin C pills," *Tufts University Health and Nutrition Letter* 18 (April 2000): 1.

37. N. Clark and colleagues, "Expert panel shuns antioxidant supplements, pushes food sources," *Environmental Nutrition* 23 (May 2000) 3; J. H. Rosenberg and colleagues, "Should you continue taking antioxidant supplements? A new, comprehensive report suggests no," *Tufts University Health and Nutrition Letter* 18 (June 2000): 1.

38. B. Liebman, "Solving the diet-and-disease puzzle," *Nutrition Action Healthletter* 26 (May 1999): 4.

39. G. Blackburn, "Whole-diet approach extends lives," *Health News* 6 (June 2000): 1.

40. F. B. Hu and colleagues, "Prospective study of major dietary patterns and risk of coronary heart disease in men," *American Journal of Clinical Nutrition* 72 (2000): 912.

14. Testing and Treatment

1. B. Zaret, M. Moses, and L. S. Cohen, *Yale University School of Medicine Heart Book* (New York: Hearst, 1992); E. J. Topol and colleagues, *Cleveland Clinic Heart Book: The Definitive Guide for the Entire Family from the Nation's Leading Heart Center* (New York: Hyperion, 2000); M. E. DeBakey and A. M. Gotto, *The New Living Heart* (Holbrook: Adams Media Corporation, 1997); N. D. Wong, H. R. Black, and J. M. Gardin, *Preventive Cardiology* (New York: McGraw Hill, 1999).

2. Topol and colleagues, *Cleveland Clinic Heart Book.*

3. T. H. Lee and colleagues, "Women and heart disease," *Harvard Heart Letter* 10 (February 2000): 1; G. S. Francis and colleagues, "How gender affects heart disease—and what you can do about it," *Cleveland Clinic Heart Advisor* 3 (February 2000): 4.

4. M. Friedman and G. J. van den Bovenkamp, "Pathogenesis of coronary thrombosis," *American Journal of Pathology,* 48 (1966): 19.

5. A. M. Gotto and H. Pownall, *Manual of Lipid Disorders: Reducing the Risk for Coronary Heart Disease,* 2nd ed. (Baltimore: Williams and Wilkins, 1999).

6. G. S. Francis and colleagues, "Statin drugs' benefits go beyond cholesterol control," *Cleveland Clinic Heart Advisor* 3 (February 2000): 3.

7. Ibid.

8. B. Jarmin, "ACE inhibitors benefit heart failure," *Journal Watch* 20 (July 1, 2000): 102.

9. Topol and colleagues, *Cleveland Clinic Heart Book.*

10. Expert Panel on Detection, Evaluation and Treatment of High Blood Cholesterol in Adults, *Journal of the American Medical Association* 285 (2001): 2486.

11. R. J. Gibbons and colleagues, "New treatment for an aching heart," *Consumer Reports on Health* 12 (February 2000): 1; R. D. Sheeler and colleagues, "Coronary stents: Tiny tubes that keep blood flowing," *Mayo Clinic Health Letter* 17 (April 1999): 1; H. C. Herrmann and colleagues, "How well do stents work?" *Heart Watch* 4 (February 2000): 1; T. H. Lee, "Angioplasty for MI should be performed within two hours," *Journal Watch* 20 (July 15, 2000): 116.

12. Gibbons and colleagues, "New treatment for an aching heart."

13. Ibid.

15. An Introduction to Cardiac Rehabilitation Programs

1. N. K. Wenger and colleagues, *Recovering from Heart Problems through Cardiac Rehabilitation: Patient Guide* (Rockville, Maryland: Agency for Health Care Policy and Research, 1995); N. K. Wenger and colleagues, *Cardiac Rehabilitation* (Rockville, Maryland: Agency for Health Care Policy and Research, 1995).

16. Cardiac Rehabilitation in Action

1. R. J. Thomas and colleagues, "National survey of gender differences in cardiac rehabilitation programs: Patient characteristics and enrollment patterns," *Cardiopulmonary Rehabilitation* 16 (1996): 402.

2. D. Louie and R. Wedell, "Exercise in a cardiac rehabilitation setting," in P. Kris-Etherton and J. H. Burns, eds., *Cardiovascular Nutrition* (American Dietetic Association, 1998), pp. 135–144; American Association of Cardiovascular and Pulmonary Rehabilitation, *Guidelines for Cardiac Rehabilitation and Secondary Prevention Programs*, 3rd ed. (Champaign, Illinois: Human Kinetics, 1995); Expert Panel on Detection, Evaluation and Treatment of High Blood Cholesterol in Adults, *Journal of the American Medical Association* 285 (2001): 2486.

3. G. Borg, *Perceived Exertion and Pain Scales* (Champaign, Illinois: Human Kinetics, 1998). Special folders can be obtained from "Borg Perception," Furuholmen 1027, 76291 Rimbo, Sweden.

4. Ibid.

5. M. Friedman, *Type A Behavior: Its Diagnosis and Treatment* (New York: Plenum, 1996); F. J. Pashkow and colleagues, "Stress kills: Controlling it could save your life," *Cleveland Clinic Heart Advisor* 2 (September 1999): 6; T. H. Lee and colleagues, "How mental stress taxes the heart," *Harvard Heart Letter* 7 (March 1997): 2; T. H. Lee and colleagues, "More on anger and heart disease," *Harvard Heart Letter* 7 (May 1997): 7.

6. D. Daniels and V. A. Price. *The Essential Enneagram: The Definitive Personality Test and Self-discovery Guide* (San Francisco: Harper, 2000).

7. Friedman, *Type A Behavior.*

8. F. J. Pashkow and colleagues, "Can spirituality make you healthier?" *Cleveland Clinic Heart Advisor* 9 (September 1998): 3.

9. V. A. Price, "Research and clinical issues in treating type A behavior." In *Type A Behavior Pattern: Research, Theory and Intervention,* ed. B. Kent-Houston and C. R. Snyder (New York: Wiley Series on Health Psychology and Behavioral Medicine, 1988), pp. 275–311.

10. P. J. Mills, "Meditation," *Science and Medicine* 6 (1999): 38.

11. H. C. Herrmann and colleagues, "Heart attack trauma," *Heart Watch* 2 (August 1998): 4; T. H. Lee and colleagues, "Emotions and heart disease," *Harvard Heart Letter* 8 (July 1998): 3; T. H. Lee and colleagues, "Grumpy old men: At risk for coronary disease?" *Harvard Heart Letter* 8 (August 1998): 7; H. C. Herrmann and colleagues, "Depression after heart attack or bypass," *Heart Watch* 3 (February 1999): 4; T. H. Lee and colleagues, "The lonely heart," *Harvard Heart Letter* 3 (December 1992): 1.

12. R. Ornstein and D. S. Sobel, *Healthy Pleasures* (Reading, Massachusetts: Perseus, 1989); A. J. Clear and S. C. Wessley, "Just what the doctor ordered—more alcohol and sex," *British Medical Journal* 315 (1997): 1638.

13. Thomas et al., "National survey of gender differences."

14. N. H. Miller and colleagues. "Home versus group exercise training for increasing functional capacity after myocardial infarction," *Circulation* 70 (1984): 645; G. F. Fletcher and colleagues, "Telephonically monitored home exercise early after coronary artery bypass surgery," *Chest* 86 (1984): 645; W. L. Haskell and colleagues, "Effects of intensive multiple risk factor reduction on coronary atherosclerosis and clinical cardiac events in men and women with coronary artery disease: The Stanford Coronary Risk Intervention Project (SCRIP)," *Circulation* 89 (1994): 975.

15. A. J. Coat and colleagues, "Effects of physical training in chronic heart failure," *Lancet* 335 (1990): 63; P. Ades and colleagues, "A controlled trial of cardiac rehabilitation in the home setting: Improving accessibility," *Journal of the American College of Cardiology* 27 (1996): 150A.

16. See note 3.

17. R. F. DeBusk and colleagues, "A case-management system for coronary risk factor modification after acute myocardial infarction," *Annals of Internal Medicine* 120 (1994): 721.

Glossary

ACE Inhibitors (Angiotensen-converting Enzymes)   Angiotensen, produced in the body, causes arteries to constrict. ACE inhibitors prevent this effect and therefore dilate the blood vessels and help lower the blood pressure. They also prolong life in people with damaged heart muscles and can help prevent heart attacks and strokes in high-risk patients.

Allergic Reaction   An abnormal reaction to a previously encountered substance introduced into the body. Manifestations may include a rash and trouble breathing.

Amino Acids   The building blocks of protein.

Anaphylaxis   Serious, potentially life-threatening allergic reaction.

Anemia   Decreased number of red blood cells; low red blood cell count.

Anesthetic   A drug or agent used to decrease or eliminate the feeling of pain. A general anesthetic puts the patient to sleep; a local anesthetic numbs an area of the body without putting the patient to sleep.

Aneurysm   A permanent dilatation of an artery, usually caused by weakening of the wall of that artery.

Angina   Any kind of discomfort or pain that occurs most commonly in the chest, but may occur in the jaw, shoulder blades, elbow, or pit of the stomach and that predictably occurs with exertion, then goes away with rest. A common symptom of coronary artery disease.

Angiogram   An invasive diagnostic test that involves placing a long catheter, often through an artery in the groin, into the origin of one of the arteries, then injecting contrast material (a solution containing an iodine compound visible on X rays) to visualize the arteries on X rays. A coronary angiogram is used to detect narrowing or blockage of the coronary arteries.

Angioplasty   An invasive procedure in which a special balloon-tipped catheter is passed into narrowed areas of the coronary artery. The balloon is then inflated, which presses the intruding plaque against the wall of the artery, dilating the inside of the artery and improving blood flow to the heart muscle.

Antihypertensive   A drug that lowers the blood pressure.

Antioxidant   A vitamin or phytochemical that is capable of counteracting the damaging effects of oxidation in tissues.

Aortic Valve   The valve located between the left ventricle and the aorta (the major artery delivering oxygenated blood to the rest of the body), which regulates blood flow between the two.

ApoE Lipoproteinemia   ApoE is a protein that comes in three versions: 2, 3, and 4. The version in any given person is inherited. The gene for ApoE is usually located on the short arm of chromosome 19, near the LDL receptor. The gene for ApoE is the one that most commonly affects the level of LDL cholesterol in the blood. People who have inherited ApoE4 have the highest LDL levels. They can significantly lower the blood levels of their LDL cholesterol by eating less saturated fat and cholesterol.

Arrhythmia   Any deviation from the normal heartbeat.

Arteriosclerosis   A thickening and hardening of the arteries; atherosclerosis is one of its forms.

Aspiration   The inhalation of fluid into the lungs through the airways.

Atherosclerosis   The development of fatty deposits in the inner lining of arteries, which then thicken the inner lining and may calcify. When this occurs, the arteries narrow. Some people develop symptoms when their arteries narrow; others do not.

Atrial Fibrillation   An arrhythmia in which the upper chambers of the heart (atria) beat very irregularly and inefficiently. The longer the atrial fibrillation lasts, the greater the risk that blood clots may form in the atria.

Atrioventricular Node   Special tissue located near the center of the heart that acts as a pacemaker and tells the ventricles when and how to beat.

Atrium A receptacle located above each ventricle. The right atrium receives blood as it returns from the rest of the body; the left atrium receives rich, oxygenated blood returning from the lungs.

Beta-Blocker (Beta-andrenegic Blocker) A medicine that blocks the action of the hormone epinephrine on the heart. Since epinephrine makes the heart beat faster and constricts small arteries, blocking the action of epinephrine lowers the heart rate, lowers the blood pressure, slows the progression of congestive heart failure, and may relieve angina.

Bile-acid Sequestrants These substances prevent the resorption of bile acids (made from cholesterol in the liver) from the bowel, thereby depleting the liver's supply of cholesterol and lowering the level of cholesterol in the blood.

Body Mass Index (BMI) A mathematical ratio between weight and height that correlates with body fat.

Bradyarrhythmia Slow, irregular heartbeat.

Bradycardia Slow heartbeat.

Bronchospasm Breathing distress caused by narrowing of the airways.

Bruce Stages Indicate the speed, measured in miles per hour (mph), and the grade of the slope (percent) at which a treadmill is set. The stages are (1) 1.7 mph at 10 percent, (2) 2.5 mph at 12 percent, (3) 3.4 mph at 14 percent, and (4) 4.2 mph at 16 percent.

Bundle Branch Block A condition in which the electric current that triggers heartbeat is obstructed between the atria and ventricles in either the right or left bundle system (a network of specialized muscle fibers in the ventricles that distribute electrical impulses originating in the atria). Changes on the EKG result, making ordinary stress tests uninformative.

Bypass Surgery See Coronary Artery Bypass Graft Surgery.

Catheter A tube for withdrawing or introducing fluids.

Chronic Bronchitis A condition in which there is continuing inflammation of the bronchial tubes.

Chronic Obstructive Pulmonary Disease   The combination of emphysema and chronic bronchitis.

Clinical Trial   An experiment utilizing human patients.

Clotbusters   See Thrombolytic Agents.

Computed Tomography (CT) Scan   Ultrafast CT is used to determine the amount of calcium present in the coronary arteries. If these arteries are not calcified, little or no coronary artery disease is present. The heavier the calcification, the worse the coronary artery disease.

Coronary Artery Bypass Graft Surgery (CABG)   A surgical procedure that involves opening the chest in order to reroute blood around a blockage in a coronary artery, using arteries or veins or both from other parts of the body.

Defibrillator   A machine capable of reestablishing normal heart rhythm by administering an electric shock to the heart externally or via a device implanted under the skin.

Diabetes   A disease characterized by excess sugar in the blood and urine. Persons with type 1 diabetes do not make insulin themselves and need insulin in order to survive. Type 2 diabetes is more common; insulin levels can be high, below normal, or normal.

Diastolic   The lower number in a blood pressure reading; pertaining to the resting or relaxation phase of the heartbeat.

Diuretic   Sometimes known as a water pill, it is a drug that causes increased urination. Lowers the blood pressure by making the kidneys excrete more sodium and water. Also used to get rid of excess water in the soft tissues of the legs and in or around the lungs in persons with congestive heart failure.

Dobutamine and Dipyridamole Stress Tests   For patients who cannot exercise, a medication (either dobutamine or dipyridamole) is used to dilate the arteries and make the heart beat rapidly. Blood flow to the heart muscle is then analyzed using either the thallium scan or an echocardiogram.

Echocardiogram   A sound wave test of the heart; see Exercise Echocardiogram.

Edema   Excess fluid.

Electrocardiogram (EKG or ECG)   Electrical tracing of the heart-beat or heart rhythm; a diagnostic test that produces a graph used for measuring electrical activity of the heart. Can become abnormal if the blood supply to the heart is inadequate.

Emphysema   A condition in which the walls of the air sacs in the lungs break down, so that they enlarge and there is an inadequate gas exchange.

Endoscopic Examination   Looking at an internal part of the body with a flexible lighted tube called an endoscope.

Exercise Echocardiogram   The use of ultrasound to evaluate the actual beating of the heart muscle before and immediately after exercise.

Factor VII   A substance in the blood that makes it clot.

Fibrates   Lower the level of triglycerides in the blood by blocking the production of triglycerides in the liver; also lower the cholesterol level in the blood.

Fibrillation   Irregular beat of the heart or other muscle.

Gastroesophageal Reflux   A phenomenon in which stomach juices flow backward up the esophagus.

HDL2   A subclass of HDL, which is divided into two further subclasses, 2a and 2b. A high level of HDL2b is beneficial because it helps to return cholesterol to the liver and unblock arteries, and because it functions as an antioxidant. Low levels increase the severity of coronary artery disease and the speed at which obstructions worsen. Low levels, which may be inherited, are associated with the small LDL disorder, syndrome X, and diabetes mellitus.

HDL3   The more dense, relatively poor subclass of HDL cholesterol. Alcohol tends to increase HDL3.

Heart Attack   Occurs when an artery feeding blood to a section of heart muscle becomes completely blocked. If the blockage lasts long enough, this section of heart muscle will die. Also called a myocardial infarction (MI).

Heart Enzymes   Proteins formed in heart cells which act as catalysts in chemical reactions. Released into the blood when heart cells die. If levels are high, the patient has had a heart attack.

Heart/Lung Machine   An apparatus that takes over the function of the heart and lungs while the heart is stopped during bypass surgery.

Hematocrit   The number of red blood cells in the blood.

Heritable Disease   A disease that can be transmitted to one's offspring and result in damage to future children.

Hiatal Hernia   A hernia of the stomach, through a small hole in the diaphragm called the hiatus.

High-density Lipoprotein (HDL, or Good Cholesterol)   The densest lipoprotein, which contains less triglyceride than any other lipoprotein and deposits cholesterol in the liver.

High-sensitivity C-reactive Protein   A marker of inflammation that can be measured in the blood. High levels seem to be the best predictor of a heart attack.

Homocysteinemia   A condition in which the blood levels of homocysteine, an amino acid, are elevated. Often, but not always, due to an inherited defect. A common cause is the abnormality of an enzyme. High levels of homocysteine in the blood cause atherosclerosis and thrombosis.

Hypoxia   Low oxygen level in the blood.

Iatrogenic   Caused by a physician or by treatment.

Idiopathic   Of unknown cause.

Indwelling   Remaining in a given location, such as a catheter.

Infarct   Death of tissue because of lack of blood supply.

Intramuscular   Into the muscle; within the muscle.

Intraperitoneal   Into the abdominal cavity.

Intravenous (IV)   Into or within a vein.

Invasive Procedure   A puncture, opening, or cutting of the skin.

Ischemia   Decreased oxygen in a tissue (usually because of decreased blood flow).

Lactovegetarian Diet   A diet that allows no meat, poultry, or fish, but does allow milk, yogurt, and cheese.

Lipid   Fat.

Lipid Profile (Panel)   Fat and cholesterol levels in the blood.

Lipoprotein   A compound made from both fat and protein.

Low-density Lipoprotein (LDL, or Bad Cholesterol)   Contains more triglyceride than HDL, is less dense, and floats more when separated out in a rapid spinning centrifuge. Deposits cholesterol onto the inner lining of the arteries, where it can form a plaque.

Lp(a)   An LDL particle with a protein called apo (a) stuck to its surface. Elevated Lp(a) is an inherited disorder; the gene is located on chromosome 6. High levels of Lp(a) are associated with heart attacks in young men. About 50 percent of the children of young men who have had a heart attack and have high levels of Lp(a) also have high levels of Lp(a) in the blood. Niacin can lower Lp(a) in men and women, as can estrogen in women.

Lumen   The cavity of an organ or tube (e.g., inside a blood vessel).

Malignancy   A cancer or other progressively enlarging and spreading tumor, fatal if not successfully treated.

Medical Foods   Used to treat a specific disease or condition.

Mitral Valve   The valve that regulates the blood flow between the left atrium and the left ventricle.

Mitral Valve Prolapse   An abnormality in which the mitral valve of the heart does not close.

Myalgia   Muscle aches.

Myocardial   Pertaining to the (muscle of the) heart.

Myocardial Infarction (MI)   Heart attack; death of the heart muscle.

Nasogastric Tube   A tube from the nose to the stomach.

Niacin   A B-complex vitamin that raises the level of HDL (good) cholesterol in the blood and lowers total cholesterol and LP(a) levels.

Noninvasive   Not breaking, cutting, or entering the skin.

Nutrient   Anything nutritious.

Occlusion   A closing or obstruction.

Osteoporosis   A bone disorder characterized by the loss of bone and leading to increased risk of fracture.

Pacemaker   A small device, implanted under the skin or worn externally, capable of reestablishing normal heart rate by administering an electric shock to the heart.

PAI-1 (Plasminogen Activator Inhibitor-1)   A substance in the bloodstream which slows the dissolution of blood clots that can cause a heart attack.

Panic Attack   Chest pain due to anxiety, not arising from the heart. In people having a panic attack, the heart pounds rapidly, they sweat, they feel short of breath or have difficulty breathing, and they feel dizzy or faint.

Phytochemicals   Plant chemicals that are neither vitamins nor minerals, and supply no calories; may have benefits for heart disease and diabetes.

Plant-based Diet   A high-fiber diet rich in phytochemicals and antioxidants, which mainly contains vegetables, whole grains, and legumes.

Plaque   A deposit of cholesterol, immune cells, muscle cells, and calcium salts in the arterial wall with a fibrous cap separating it from the blood.

Pleuritis   An inflammation of the sac covering the lungs, which can cause a sharp pain in the chest with every breath.

Restenosis   The formation of scar tissue after angioplasty or by-pass surgery, which may cause as much or more narrowing than existed before the procedure.

Saturated Fat   A type of single-bond animal or vegetable fat that increases LDL cholesterol levels in blood.

Shingles   A disease caused by the chicken pox virus, which generates severe pain.

Sinoatrial Node (Sinus Node)   Special tissue located in the right atrium that acts as a pacemaker and tells the heart when and how to beat.

Sludging   A phenomenon in which red cells tend to clump together as they pass through very small arteries.

Small, Dense LDL Particles   LDL particles are spheres that come in a wide range of sizes and densities. Everyone has both large and small LDL particles in their blood. Existing coronary artery disease progresses twice as fast in patients with a high proportion of small, dense LDL particles, as compared to those with mostly large, buoyant ones. The gene for small, dense LDL particles is located on the short arm of chromosome 19, near the LDL receptor.

Sonogram A graphic outline of the heart's movement, created through high-frequency sound waves.

Statin Drugs (HMG-CoA Reductive Inhibitors) Medications that block the production of cholesterol in the liver. They also relax the muscles in the walls of the arteries, preventing the arteries from going into spasm, and reduce inflammation in plaques, preventing them from rupturing.

Stenosis Abnormal narrowing of an artery or heart valve.

Stent A special metal scaffolding inserted after balloon angioplasty to keep the artery dilated.

Syndrome A group of symptoms that together are characteristic of a specific condition.

Syndrome X Characterized by elevated blood triglycerides, low HDL cholesterol, slow clearance of fat from the blood, small, dense LDL cholesterol particles, excess fibrinogen in the blood, excess PAI-1, and high blood pressure.

Systolic The upper number in a blood pressure reading; pertaining to the contraction phase of the heartbeat.

Telemetry A method or device for transmitting data about heart rhythm to a remote television screen.

Thallium Exercise Test The injection of radioactive thallium into a vein, which outlines the portion of the heart muscle receiving inadequate blood flow during exercise.

Thrombolytic Agents (Clotbusters) Medications administered soon after a heart attack to break up the clot that caused the attack.

Thrombosis Blood clotting within blood vessels.

Toxicity Undesirable reaction or side effects of a drug.

Trans Fats Created by converting vegetable oil to a solid or semi-solid margarine through a process known as hydrogenation.

Treadmill Exercise Test A test that involves walking on a machine used to determine heart function. As the speed of the treadmill and its incline increase, any symptoms, as well as the pulse rate, blood pressure, and electrocardiogram, are monitored.

Triglycerides (Blood Fat)   Three fatty acids attached to a glycerol molecule.

Vasospasm   A narrowing of the blood vessels due to a spasm of the vessel walls.

Vegan Diet   Based on whole grains, legumes, and vegetables, which contains no animal products whatsoever.

Ventricles   The pumping chambers of the heart, located below each atrium.

Ventricular Fibrillation   An arrhythmia in which the ventricles of the heart beat weakly and irregularly.

Ventricular Tachycardia   A condition in which the ventricles beat very rapidly, independently of the atria.

Very Low-Density Lipoprotein (VLDL)   A lipoprotein that contains more triglycerides than any other lipoprotein; the least dense lipoprotein, which floats when separated out in a rapidly spinning centrifuge.

Contributors

Health Professionals

Kathleen Berra, M.S.N., A.N.P., F.A.A.C.V.P.R., F.A.A.N., cofounded one of the first community-based cardiac rehabilitation programs in the United States. She was a founding member of the American Association of Cardiovascular and Pulmonary Rehabilitation, serving as its second president, and is currently editor-in-chief of the *Journal of Cardiopulmonary Rehabilitation* and clinical trial director of the Stanford Center for Research in Disease Prevention.

Gerald W. Friedland, M.D., is professor emeritus of radiology at Stanford University. He graduated from medical school forty-six years ago. After his internship, Dr. Friedland trained for three years in internal medicine, with a year each of cardiology and gastroenterology. He passed the membership examination of the Royal College of Physicians of Edinburgh with gastroenterology his subspecialty; he was later elected a fellow of the college. He subsequently trained in radiology, where he focused on gastrointestinal, urinary, and pediatric radiology.

Christopher Gardner, PH.D., is an assistant professor at the Stanford Center for Research in Disease Prevention, where he is director of nutrition studies. He has conducted several clinical trials that examined the potential benefits of various dietary components and of vegetarian diets on risk factors for heart disease among adults with elevated risk profiles.

Francis H. Koch, M.D., F.A.C.C., is medical consultant to the Cardiac Therapy Foundation of the Midpeninsula in Palo Alto, California. He received his medical degree from Cornell University in 1969, then served as an intern at the New York Hospital–Cornell Medical Center, and later as a resident there in internal medicine. Dr. Koch trained in cardiology at the Stanford University School of Medicine, where he was appointed clinical professor of medicine (cardiology). He has a private practice in Palo Alto.

Donna Louie, R.N., B.S.N., is program director of the Cardiac Therapy Foundation of the Midpeninsula and has worked in all phases of cardiac rehabilitation for the last sixteen years. She served on the board of directors of the California Society for Cardiac Rehabilitation, and was president of its northern region.

Nancy Houston Miller, R.N., B.S.N., F.A.A.C.V.P.R., is associate director of the Stanford Cardiac Rehabilitation Program, and adjunct clinical assistant professor at the University of California San Francisco School of Nursing. She has staffed classes at the Cardiac Therapy Foundation of the Midpeninsula for twenty-seven years. A past chair of the board of the California affiliate of the American Heart Association, she has served on the national board of directors of the AHA and is a cofounder and past chair of the Lipid Nurse Task Force.

Barton Thurber, PH.D., is professor of English at the University of San Diego. After his undergraduate work at Stanford University, he worked for two years as a medical research assistant at the university's School of Medicine. He received his graduate degree from Harvard University. Thurber has published more than fifty papers in his field; has had a play produced in New York; has written, coedited, or edited thirty-six medical articles; is the editor of a medical textbook; and has worked in the fields of psychology, biochemistry, and behavior management.

Robin Wedell, R.N., B.S.N., is program associate director of the Cardiac Therapy Foundation of the Midpeninsula and has worked in all phases of cardiac rehabilitation for the last thirteen years. With Donna Louie (see above) she wrote "Exercise in a Cardiac Rehabilitation Setting" in *Cardiovascular Nutrition.*

Participants

Sonny Adams	Max Kramer
Hans Forsell	Helen L'Amoreaux
Jerry Fox	David Moses
Jacob Gershon	Verne Peters
Jose Ibarra	Joy Sing
Peter Jones	

Index